AF679278

The Spark Within

LIVING LIFE with AUTOIMMUNE DISEASES

Samantha Smith

Grosvenor House Publishing Limited

This book is published by
Grosvenor House Publishing Ltd
Link House
140 The Broadway, Tolworth, Surrey, KT6 7HT.
www.grosvenorhousepublishing.co.uk

A CIP record for this book
is available from the British Library

Paperback ISBN 978-1-83615-450-1

What a journey it's been so far. As a woman with three diagnosed autoimmune conditions before the age of 35, I have had quite the ride through life. From the teenage years onwards, I have known nothing of life without a medical condition and all that comes with it. But do you know what? I have lived! And you can too!

If you feel alone or don't know how to relate to someone who has just received an autoimmune diagnosis, I hope my experiences can help you understand one key fact: after a low, there always comes a high!

The Spark Within:
Living Life with Autoimmune Diseases xx

This book is dedicated to my husband, mum, brother, late grandparents, best friend and dog.

They are the ones that have had my back all throughout my life, who have listened over the years and shook their heads in disbelief at my stories. The ones that pick me up on my darker days and allow me to run with my crazy ideas on others. They have always acknowledged that things can be hard for me but have come along for the ride all the same.

There is nothing I can do to repay you all.

xxx

This is also for all the autoimmune warriors, their families and their support networks everywhere. I hope that, by sharing my experiences, I can help you to feel less alone.

xxx

Please note I am not a medical practitioner; all the ideas are drawn from my own experiences and understanding of autoimmune conditions, built up from my personal research and living experience of life with them. Always consult a doctor about your own personal circumstances.

CONTENTS

Chapter One: Diabetes Diaries 1

Chapter Two: The Grieving Process 14

Chapter Three: Hypos and Happiness 20

Chapter Four: Carbs are not the Enemy 26

Chapter Five: Insulin Pump vs MDI 35

Chapter Six: POI 41

Chapter Seven: Coeliac Disease 49

Chapter Eight: Live Your Dreams 62

Favourite Recipes 73

Chapter One: Diabetes Diaries

I have always been a foodie, challenging the appetites of my uncles and Grandad every Christmas. I was the first to opt for having two servings of pud and happy to help in the kitchen whenever I could.

Coming home from school to a chicken roast dinner on a Wednesday was the first time I realised something was wrong. Mum never cooked midweek roasts and all I could think of as I looked at the piled plate was 'I can't eat it'.

The following week I was sat in a German lesson, a year seven student still finding her way, when I came over really dizzy and felt sick. I was excused from class and went to the receptionist who called my mum to pick me up. I remember sitting with my then best friend sipping a 'Volvic Touch of Fruit' – flavoured water packed with sugar – from the strawberry syrup, which made it taste delicious compared to plain old boring tap water.

When Mum arrived, she said we were going to the doctors', but I begged her to just take me home. I lost the argument and we managed to get an appointment at the doctors' pretty much immediately. Little did I know that would be the last drink I would ever have without a care in the world.

We sat in the waiting room, waves of sickness washing over me. I had this unbelievable exhaustion which made me feel like curling up in a ball in the corner and sleeping for a week.

A quick blood test via a finger prick led to a pretty dismissive 'she's got diabetes, you had better head to the hospital' diagnosis directed straight at my mum. There was no explanation, no addressing me, just a direct instruction for us to go. Next thing I knew, I was slumped in the back of Mum's car. We picked up my Aunty enroute and I was rushed into the Children's ward of the hospital in the nearest city. I remember the colourful hospital ward walls, the horrible smell of the food cooking and the look of panic on everyone's face.

The rest of that afternoon was a blur.

Later on that day, I remember standing on the scales feeling frail and exhausted. I weighed 6.5 stone despite my already tall 5ft 8in frame. On reflection, that Volvic water did absolutely nothing to quench my thirst. The thirst was just unreal; drinking endless water, tea, coffee or fizzy pop, nothing made me feel even remotely hydrated. I had been going to the toilet more often and, it was fair to say, my body was absolutely exhausted – I was so tired all the time.

There are so many misconceptions and assumptions about diabetes and diabetics. It really is very difficult to put into words for a non-diabetic what this condition really entails. I am not a qualified medic and everyone who has diabetes or knows someone with diabetes should research the condition for their own benefit. If this is your first stop on your diabetes education tour, then here's some basics on the science:

Diabetes is an autoimmune condition which occurs when the pancreas does not produce enough of the hormone insulin or the body cannot effectively use the insulin it creates. Insulin is the hormone which regulates blood sugar, and for type one diabetes, insulin is used as the only form of treatment.

There are several different types of diabetes: type one, type two, gestational, monogenic diabetes, cystic-fibrosis diabetes, type 3c, Latent Autoimmune Disease in Adults (LADA) and Maturity Onset Diabetes of the Young (MODY).

Each and every type of diabetes comes with its own challenges and no two diabetics are the same. A diabetes diagnosis is very much a condition that tends to come up and bite the person diagnosed with it when they least expect it.

The four key signs of diabetes are:

1. Thin – losing a lot of weight
2. Thirst – drinking a lot more fluids
3. Toilet – going to the toilet more frequently
4. Tired – always feeling exhausted

Please, please, please, if you recognise any of the '4 T's' in yourself or a friend or loved one, make sure to get to the doctors' as soon as possible. You could save a life.

As the day of my diagnosis turned into night, the Nurses tried to get me to eat something. I remember having two bits of white bread toast and watching Red Dwarf II. I can't remember a single thing about the episode, but I do remember that trying to eat two bits of stale toast whilst having a drip in each arm was a bit of a challenge. There was this eerie quietness about the ward that night as I lay alone waiting for the morning to come back round.

Over the next few days, I had a few visitors, friends, family, all coming through the door with the same look of despair that I had seen when I entered the ward. There were coming and goings by different doctors, consultants and nurses. On my second night, I cried. Overtired and overwhelmed, I was comforted by the best diabetes specialist nurse I have ever come across in over twenty years as a diabetic; she had type one too. She is the only nurse I have spoken to that truly 'got it'. She sat on my bed and we talked and cried together. She explained how she cared about diabetics and her own experiences throughout her life. We spoke for a long time about life aspirations. I shared what I wanted to be when I grew up, what my plans were after school, and she reassured me that all of it was still possible with diabetes (even though it didn't feel like it then!). I will be forever grateful to that nurse; she set up for a lifetime of resilience with this challenging disease.

The next step in my somewhat whirlwind education on how to keep myself alive was to learn how to inject myself. The nurses were quite clear that I would not be allowed home until they were confident I could do injections by myself. That's when they presented me with… an orange. The reason? Because 'the peel is like human skin'. I can honestly say I have never looked at an orange the same way again.

Thankfully, I was a kid who was not fazed by needles. I was shown how to load an insulin cartridge into the pen, attach a needle, squirt out an air shot and then pinch the skin to inject. On an orange that is. I cannot remember the first injection I did to myself. Everyone seems to think the injections are the hard part of living with diabetes, but really they just become part of the new lifestyle routine, a habit even. To put things in perspective, I have injected myself for over 8,000 consecutive days now with an understanding that I will likely need to do this forever and there are maybe two or three injections I remember. Either because they hurt or were awkward!

One of the most important elements of diabetes management is blood sugar testing. Throughout my time in hospital, my fingers were pricked and blood sugars tested every hour.

In the early days, the only way of testing your blood sugars was by pricking your finger with a lancet loaded into a pull-back spring pen and placing a droplet of blood right in the middle of a testing strip which was then inserted into a chunky machine. You had to wait through a 20 second countdown before seeing the result flash on the screen.

The optimal blood sugar reading is 4-7 mmol. Higher than 7 and you are considered hyperglycemic and lower than 4 you are hypoglycemic. Now that's a great target, but wow is it tough to stay within that range every day.

When I was first diagnosed, the expectation was that I would test my blood sugar in the morning and in the evening. Over the next couple of years this increased to before every mealtime and before bed. Here we are in 2026 with continuous glucose monitors that track our sugars 24/7.

That weighs heavy. We have gone from a little bit of data to constant data feeds. For a diabetic, data is a tool for management but the toll of being able to know how life affects blood sugar readings every moment of everyday is a lot. Sometimes a little too much. Back when I was a newly diagnosed teenager there were times I would resent testing my sugar levels. If I had eaten something sweet and knew they were going to be elevated, there would be this almost underlying anxiety about the number on the screen not being perfect. As the years have gone by, I have learnt to understand that it's impossible to be perfect all the time with diabetes management and the most I can do is try. I do feel for the newly diagnosed as I remember the endless pressure to only have perfect readings, without any compassion for those moments when they are not in that sweet 4-7 mmol range.

As I sat in the hospital, anxious to get home to normal life, I remember the hospital teacher coming to the bedside and saying 'you have at least two hours until the doctor will come and discharge you so you'd better come to school'. I looked at Mum, she looked at me, burst out laughing and told me I had better go to school! I couldn't believe it. I sat on a tiny plastic chair next to a five-year-old, staring at the door and wishing away the next couple of hours.

Mum and I had a lot of information to absorb in those few days. We were told not to prick the top of my fingers when doing a blood test as I could go blind in later life and need my fingertips to read brail. There was a huge list of dos and don'ts around food: don't eat too much sugar but do eat carbs at every meal, don't eat chocolate unless it's after a main meal for easy absorption, be careful of PE at school because your blood sugars will drop unless you eat sugar before. There was an absolute minefield of information that would make the newly diagnosed diabetics cringe today.

We were told to expect me to be in 'the honeymoon period' for up to eighteen months post diagnosis. This is when your pancreas may still be producing minimal amounts of insulin, so dosage via injection might remain at reduced levels. In time, newly diagnosed diabetics are prone to finding their blood sugars becoming more erratic and that will mean that insulin will need to increase as their pancreas starts to give up completely.

I sat on the end of the bed, waiting to be discharged whilst I watched the London Marathon on the television, and thought to myself: 'I am going to run that one day'.

A type one diabetes diagnosis rocks your world – and not in a good way. The life you once knew is ripped from beneath you and you feel alone. Nobody in my family had suffered with diabetes so we knew nothing about the condition or what managing it entailed.

That being said, if you are reading this as a newly diagnosed diabetic or a loved one of a newly diagnosed diabetic, I promise you it gets easier. Injecting and blood sugar testing becomes second nature. Although it might seem like you are in a very dark place now, there is light. The research is coming on leaps and bounds and the advancements in treatment are making this condition so much easier to manage day-to-day. Hang in there: I promise it will get better!

I spent a total of five days in the intensive care unit, finger pricks all throughout the night, drips, endless faces of sorrow coming in through the door muttering 'are you OK? Do you have any questions?' Then I was flung back into the real world as a walking, talking pancreas, responsible for keeping myself alive every second of everyday for, well, forever.

After being discharged from hospital, I was told to go back to school the following week. I had secured a place at my first choice of secondary school in my ambition to become a solicitor. It was an all-girls school, which came with its own challenges. As a year seven student with a rucksack two thirds the size of me and a plait

I could sit on, the last thing I wanted was another thing to draw attention to myself.

Mum dropped me back to school the first day, rather than me having to catch the bus. I was armed with a Tupperware box full of mini cans of Coca Cola, biscuits and dextrose tablets. It had 'Samantha's Hypo Box' firmly attached to the front. We dropped off the box at reception and Mum explained to the friendly receptionist that, if my blood sugars fell too low, then I had to be given that box to treat it. That was followed by a big hug and a nervous smile from Mum and then I was thrown back into the wilderness of secondary school with a chronic incurable disease.

We all had to sit in alphabetical order in our form rooms. The form tutor would stand at the front and relay any school messages and important information. On my very first day back at school, guess who was the topic of the form discussion? I wanted the ground to swallow me up. I sat on the second row and I could feel the heads turning and eyes burning into the back of my head whilst the tutor explained that, if I felt funny, I might need to leave the classroom and go to my box in reception. It was all very surreal. I had never been a popular kid at school, but my diagnosis did lead to some people showing a bit of an interest in my condition. Thinking back to those early years, nobody around me had an aunty, grandma or cat with diabetes, unlike today where everyone seems to know someone.

Retinal eye screening. The annual appointment that no diabetic really looks forward to. I was scheduled in for my first review pretty soon after my diagnosis. Back in those early days, a specialist 'eye screening unit' (a converted bus!) used to park up in the doctor's car park to schedule in all the diabetics for their check-up.

The eye screening appointment involved a short sight test and then some eyedrops being inserted into both eyes to dilute the pupils ready for the scan. The drops burn for all of two seconds before you can blink again freely. You are sent to the waiting room to sit for ten minutes whilst the eyedrops take effect. During that ten minutes your eyesight becomes a little blurred (no scrolling Instagram!) and your eyes become a little sensitive to the light. For very good reason you are not allowed to drive after the retinal screening appointment, and you are always advised to bring sunglasses for afterwards.

The scan itself is just like a trip to the opticians; you look down the lens and stare at the green dot. A bright flash of light and a photograph of the back of your eye appears on the screen. Vision remains a little blurry for a couple of hours after the appointment but then you are right back to normal. A letter comes through (it used to be by post but now it's digital) with your results within two weeks or so.

I remember the first time seeing the retinal screening images and thinking they looked like a picture of Mars: red and orange with no sign of life!

Over the years, my results remained clear until the letter fell through the letterbox confirming I had signs of background retinopathy. This is when there are signs of damage to the blood vessels at the back of your eyes. It was 'an inevitable part of having diabetes for over ten years', I was told by a doctor.

As well as hospital clinic appointments, GPs will often want to see a diabetic separately to assess prescription requirements. Unfortunately, my experience has been that the two paths do not meet no matter how hard you try. Left and right arm do not speak to one another. A diabetic review at the doctor's surgery usually involves a consultation with either the Practice Diabetes Nurse or a GP. The format is usually weight, height and blood pressure followed by a very generic discussion around blood sugar control. There are usually no exchanges of advice around insulin dosage or practical management of diabetes; it's more of a check that you have contact with the diabetes clinic at the hospital. The diabetic review does serve a purpose insofar as it means there is a checkpoint to make sure you have all the medicines you require, any adjustments to medication volume requirements can be made there and then.

At the doctor's surgery review appointments, I had my feet checked. As a diabetic we hear horror stories of amputations for those who had not managed their blood sugars over the years. Diabetes complications are something that I try not to think about, in all honesty, and I very much have the attitude of 'I can only try my best'. Numbness or pain in feet and hands of diabetics is usually the first sign that something is up. The doctors use a piece of plastic, which is a bit like a fibre optic tube, to point to different areas of your feet and you simply have to say 'yes' if you can feel it. They usually also use an ultrasound machine to check blood flow.

I am sceptical about diabetes advice from those who are not diabetic themselves, doctors included. Unfortunately, there is only one person who can determine life's course with this condition – you. Doctors can read textbooks, attend seminars and compare you against the patient they spoke to in the appointment twenty minutes before yours, but they have no experience of your life, your job, your family demands, your hobbies or your food preferences. They cannot and should not be treating you as 'just another diabetic'.

Over the years I have sometimes become very frustrated with medical teams who do not seem to acknowledge what this disease entails. As a kid I used to have to record all my blood sugar readings in my monitoring book – this was way before the diabetes clinic could access the CGM portal and see it all – and the doctor would say 'why were your levels at 18 mmols on the 25th August?' and expect me to be able to recite exactly what I had eaten that day to make my blood sugars react in such a way.

Ignorance is something you come to tolerate as a diabetic. We should not have to but unfortunately you come to brace yourself for comments like: 'I could never inject myself every day. I would rather die!' from people that just do not get it. As a diabetic, you will find yourself become more and more resilient to people's thoughtless perceptions and comments around your condition and, in time, you will probably smile to yourself about just how idiotic some people's comments can be.

For those of us with type one diabetes, the truth is that insulin is the only thing keeping us alive. Do we want to inject ourselves multiple times a day? No. Do we want to die? No. Keep going, you got this.

The annual diabetes clinic appointment used to be a draining, constant criticism of Hba1C results. The Hba1C blood test is still used as a measure of assessing the control of diabetes across a three-month period, though more focus is placed on 'time in range' than overall Hba1C these days. In my adult years, I remember an appointment where my time in range was 52% for the 30-day period before and the nurse telling me that was 'good'. I have always been highly critical of my control and, to me, a medical professional telling me that my body functioning as it should for only 50% of a month was 'good' was shocking. But that shock incites a huge drive in me to do better. I am not perfect, far from it. I love food, I love a glass of fizz and some days the thought of picking up the dumbbells and doing a workout really does not appeal, but I have to make sure I am in range for at least 70% of the time; I can at least be three-quarters normal, right?

Chapter Two: The Grieving Process

There is a profound sense of grief you feel for the life you knew. I think that's the hardest thing for someone with auto-immune conditions to communicate: how it feels, not just the physical impact but the emotional effect a diagnosis has on you.

I was 12 when I was diagnosed as diabetic.

I remember a life where I could get up in the morning, eat a bowl of coco pops, run around the playground at school, go around my friend's for pizza and stay up 'til the early hours talking without ever having to think about a blood sugar reading or injection.

I remember being able to scoff two servings of my nan's delicious cakes without a care in the world.

I remember being able to get excited for a day out with a picnic without having to consider what time we would be eating and whether I needed to pack snacks to prevent a hypo.

I remember being able to leave the house with nothing but the house key and not having to take out a huge bag of medical supplies.

I was 33 when I was diagnosed as coeliac.

I remember the taste of freshly baked bread from the bakery cut into thick slices and eaten whilst it was still warm.

I remember the 'McDonald's treat' on a Saturday.

I remember when I used to cook Christmas dinner without fearing that someone would hate the gluten free version or having to guard against cross-contamination.

Grief is defined as 'a feeling of great sadness'. We often think of grief when someone we love dies or someone 'grieving' the loss of a person that mattered to them. In a way, when you get a life-changing illness you do grieve your old self. You lose yourself for a little while whilst you adjust to your new-normal. You look at life through a whole new lens. One of gratitude tinged with a little sadness. You reflect, you worry, and you think a lot about what the future holds.

I have always been a 'look forwards not backwards' person, but do you know what? Sometimes, I do look backwards... because I am human. Anyone who has been given a diagnosis which changes their life will feel an emptiness around the life they once knew. They might not wallow in it but there is a feeling of sadness. Just a fleeting memory of something that once was but can't be anymore.

For me, I often find myself staring longingly at people eating food I wish I could eat. I ask to smell my husband's food sometimes so I can partake in at least some of the experience of different food choices.

When I think about my life as a 12-year old and look at those who are 12 today, I do not know how I coped. Children have this utterly brilliant resilience to things that would crush an adult. I don't know how I can ever repay my mum for managing it all so brilliantly.

When I was first diagnosed, I knew of nobody else who was living with type one diabetes. Social media wasn't a thing and the only time I ever saw other diabetics was when I went to the diabetes clinic and sat in the waiting room. I remember meeting a family whose toddler had been diagnosed at the age of two and the parents sat talking to Mum for a while. I remember thinking: 'That poor kid; they are never going to remember a life without this condition.'

Throughout my teenage years, diabetes sucked. It was something that made me different to everyone else. Whilst my friends were out living care-free lives, drinking, eating, finding boys, I spent a lot of time battling high and low blood sugars, trying to understand how I was supposed to live with this illness forever.

Diabetes burnout is common amongst diabetics. It is a term that I have only really heard used over the past ten years or so, but it is essentially when you lose interest in managing your diabetes altogether. This is so closely linked to the 'grief' I am referring to in this chapter.

Decision fatigue affects us all in different ways. The first thing I think of when I wake up is my blood sugar. If I have a headache, my automatic assumption is my blood sugars must have been low overnight. If I wake up busting for the toilet, I automatically think it must be because my blood sugars are high. When I wake up and administer my first injection of the day, my maths calculations begin. I have to think about what my current blood sugar reading is, what I am going to eat for breakfast and at what time, how active I am going to be for the four hours following my breakfast as well as: how I am feeling, whether I have any stressful meetings planned, whether it is my time of the month, what the weather is outside…

If I am in a meeting or on a Teams call and can feel my blood sugars dropping, I have to make decisions. When I need to commute to an office three hours away from home, I have to plan and schedule blood tests, snack breaks and insulin to make sure my insurance covers my journey (blood sugars have to be over 5 mmol to drive) and that I have sufficient time to get to where I need to be without my diabetes getting in the way. When I have a girls' day out scheduled, I have to plan how I am going to ensure my blood sugars remain stable for the entire day. I also have to make sure that I pack enough medical supplies and I will need to make sure the group has thought about food and the timings of it. I constantly have to make sure I have enough medicine prescribed, ordered and ready to literally keep myself alive every day.

Every single day in the life of a diabetic requires countless, potential life-changing decisions, if we get something wrong.

For parents managing the blood sugars of their little ones, they are bearing this mental load on their child's behalf. They are the ones that society expects to function as a normal human being whilst being riddled with concern that their child is out of their sight and might suffer from a hypo and fall into a coma.

As a teenager, I tried to fit in with everyone else but struggled. I was not in the cool crew, but I did have a close group of friends. They would all look out for me if my levels dropped low or I had a bad day and needed to vent. That all changed when I hit sixth form and our friendship group disbanded; people changed and everyone went on their own path to find their way in the world.

As an adult, I realised a few years ago that I wake up every morning and check that I can still feel my feet by wiggling my toes. Can you imagine that? Subconsciously having a fear that you are going to lose limbs so waking up in the morning, checking your blood sugar and wiggling your toes becomes routine. Bonkers. But this is reality for a lot of us. We are surrounded by a society which is plagued with misconceptions about autoimmune conditions. Our bodies feel what our mind thinks and when you are surrounded by 'amputations because of diabetes' news stories that is what your mind and body reacts to, even if only subconsciously.

Grief does not just affect the person diagnosed with an autoimmune condition; it hurts those around them too. My whole family was rocked by my diagnosis, and I noticed a change in some of my friends too. A lot of families blame themselves, thinking it's 'genetics', but in truth it is just the card dealt. I have noticed in my older years that there is so little support for those families affected by diabetes that the feeling of isolation must be terrifying. My poor mum did not have social media to go to for answers back when I was diagnosed. There were no 'parents of diabetics' support groups' and there were absolutely no other parents (or kids!) we knew going through the same thing.

Grief is not the same for everyone. Some people will not look at their diagnosis and acknowledge that it is a traumatic event, although some will. Others will look back and realise their diagnosis was a blessing in disguise, leading them to lead a healthier life, whilst some will resent it forever. No two diabetics experiences are the same and nobody should be expected to manage their condition in the same way as another. The beauty of being a human is that we are all uniquely different, we all know ourselves better than anyone else.

Chapter Three: Hypos and Happiness

A hypo or 'hypoglycemia' occurs when your body does not have enough sugar. There are many symptoms of a hypo: sweating, confusion, shaking and unconsciousness. Hypos are extremely serious and can lead to a diabetic person falling into a coma if not treated quickly or efficiently.

Hypos can be scary. No two are the same, and when first diagnosed, you have no idea what to expect. Once you have had your first hypo you think you know, but you don't for several years. A hypo can strike any time and be a result of too much insulin, not enough food, stress, illness and around a hundred other variables.

It is so important for diabetics to check their blood sugar levels frequently to try and catch hypos quickly. Over my years as a diabetic, I have had a fair few hypos, many of which have provided entertainment (in hindsight!) to friends and family.

I remember an occasion at school where I was physically escorted out of the canteen for becoming aggressive when the dinner lady would not accept my plastic folder of notes from my previous lesson as payment for my sausages and jacket potato. I was taken straight to the medical room where I tested my sugars and found I had low sugars, below 4mmol. I had some dextrose tablets and a snack and felt more like myself around fifteen minutes later.

Whilst studying for my GCSEs I had a really rough time with my sugar levels. In hindsight, I think there was a lot more going on in my body, with an hormonal imbalance also contributing, but at the time I was none-the-wiser. We would be sat in alphabetical order as we had to in all our classes and I would feel myself nodding off and then coming back to. People must have noticed, but nobody said anything until the school called my mum and told her. That's the first time I remember being embarrassed of diabetes. My natural reaction was to block it out and pretend nothing was happening. In reality, my body was utterly exhausted from the rollercoaster ride that sugars provided, so much so that I couldn't concentrate.

There is a lot of shame that comes from hypos. That lack of control and awareness can make you feel a little embarrassed, particularly through those teenage years. The symptoms of a hypo can mean you get confused for being drunk, which is obviously a huge issue when out socialising in your late teens.

Recovering from a hypo is not instant. It can take 45 minutes for your brain and body to fully recover. After a hypo, you feel tired and lethargic. It can take a while to feel like yourself again, particularly if you have had a hypo in your sleep overnight. It is something that you should not ever feel ashamed about. There have been times I have dragged myself to work after a night of consistent lows, feeling worn out, emotional and with the classic 'hypo headache'. For what? To try and prove I was the same as everyone else. The truth is that I am not. Health has to come first and, to be honest, you should be completely honest with your employer around any allowances you need for your diabetes care.

There were a few times in the early days of finding alcohol that I took diabetes a little too close to the wire, going out for wine without eating enough and mixing drinks meant that diabetes smacked me in the face a couple of times. I quickly learnt that I could not get away with pushing my body to the limits other people seemed to get away with, and nor did I want to. Alcohol causes your blood sugar to drop in most cases. This means whenever a diabetic is planning on having a couple of drinks, they need to effortlessly plan their food, insulin and exercise around their alcohol consumption so as not to cruise through the evening fighting low blood sugars.

As I entered adulthood and my career started progressing, my role became global, and I managed a team all across the world. Different time zones meant meetings would be planned outside of normal routines. It also meant I was expected to travel and, as a senior leader, attend corporate events. This only increased the apprehension I feel towards solo travel with diabetes. My husband and I love travelling and would happily hop around the globe if it paid. The first time I had to catch a flight by myself my usually independent self needed a kick up the backside. I was not travelling with any colleagues, so I really was a lone ranger. My husband has my CGM app linked to his phone and, over the four days I was away, I would get texts: 'are you sorting your levels?', 'what have you got for dinner?'. Those messages mean the world to a diabetic and reassure you that you are not alone in the fight.

For me trusting my body can be a bit of a struggle sometimes. For many years it felt like we were fighting each other and with that comes a lack of trust. When you are responsible for the work of an organ, you have got to do what you need to so you can maintain as much control as possible.

The top hypo that will go down in our family history was at my nan and grandad's house during the school holidays. I had let my sugars go low to the point I was completely disorientated. I told my nan I was going to the toilet, only to go into their kitchen, pick up the teapot and try and get into their pantry cupboard. I remember Nan rushing through the kitchen door, grabbing the teapot and pushing me down to the floor. Grandad tried to come in to find out what was going on only to be ushered back into the hallway.

My nan never quite accepted my diabetes diagnosis, or 'sugar diabetes' as she would call it. My nan and grandad lived the good life: they didn't have corporate careers, they had a modest house they bought from the Council, and they loved each other dearly. They would eat breakfast, lunch and dinner together every day. At 10am it was time for a couple of biscuits with a cup of tea and at 3pm they either had a scone or one of Nan's home-baked delicious cakes came out with the afternoon cup of tea. My brother and I would spend the school holidays with our grandparents and would love baking (and eating) all the delicious treats they would spoil us with.

During the first school holidays following my diagnosis, Nan suggested we have a go at baking a low sugar cake. We went to Sainsbury's and stocked up on powdered sweetener ready to tackle the challenge. Nan was a fantastic baker, everyone loved her cakes, especially her Victoria sponge and fruit scones. Every sweet treat was homemade and she took real pride in the family enjoying her bakes, as I do now.

We whisked up the cake mix and put it in the oven, with everything crossed for a successful bake. I still remember Nan's disappointment when the sponge came out of the oven, flat as a pancake. She was absolutely mortified. I was just grateful to have cake and happily ate it even though Nan was totally mortified she hadn't created a 5* masterpiece.

Unfortunately, hypos are part and parcel of a diabetes diagnosis. There are lots of things to balance and weigh up whilst managing this illness and one thing that really is important is having hypo awareness. This means being able to recognise the signs of a hypo coming on so you can act fast and bring those blood sugars up quickly.

In the UK, a type one diabetic needs to apply for their driving licence every three years. On each application, a health declaration has to be made that nothing has changed with the illness that could impact upon our driving ability. No awareness of hypos is a serious issue when it comes to driving – even if you don't 'feel' it, your body is lacking the energy required to function properly and that means you are potentially a danger behind the wheel.

Lots of things can affect hypo awareness, including suffering through a really severe hypo, running blood sugars too high or too low, or sometimes awareness is just lost for no reason. It is really important to monitor your blood sugars closely so, even if you do not feel funny, you know when you need to take action.

As a diabetic, it is hugely important to have a network of family and friends you can literally trust with your life. I tend to portray myself as a 'strong and independent woman' but, in reality, I would be absolutely lost without those I love; they have helped me battle all the highs and lows the past 30 odd years.

Chapter Four: Carbs are not the Enemy

The recommended diet as a diabetic back at my time of diagnosis was completely different to what we are all told today. Historically, the advice was carbohydrates at each meal, a little fun-size chocolate bar before PE and a maximum of three bags of crisps a week was my favourite...

During my time in hospital, Mum and I put together a list of foods which we asked whether I would still be able to have in this new world as a diabetic: Sunny D, Mr Frosty Cola Pops, Jaffa Cakes (tell me you're a 90s kid without telling me you're a 90s kid!). There was so much focus on what you could not eat rather than what you should be eating.

At each clinic appointment, diabetes nurse appointment or GP visit for a prescription review, my weight was always taken. Regardless of the appointment context, weight was always the number one job. There was one diabetes nurse visit where the nurse gasped at my weight as I stood on the scales, which has stuck with me forever.

When someone is diagnosed with a chronic illness they already carry the burden of 'living a healthy life' on their shoulders. You ask yourself 'why me?', 'was there anything I could have done?', 'maybe it was the chocolate muffin I had that tipped me over the edge?' All sorts of thoughts and questions are left to whizz around your head. The last thing a person needs is for a doctor, nurse or anyone else in fact to tell them that they need to be mindful of their weight when they are nowhere near tracking as overweight or obese for their height and frame.

From that appointment on, I started independently researching more about diabetes. I would read articles and forums where diabetics would say following a low-carb diet changed their life, making their blood sugar more manageable and their waistline shrink. I jumped on the bandwagon in my late teens and, sure enough, the weight dropped off. My blood sugars became a little more manageable in the short-term, until they weren't. I had no energy, I was hungry, and I really fancied some crisps!

You might not be aware, but under data protection law, you have the right to request your own medical records under a 'subject access request'. After twenty years of managing diabetes and being hit with other diagnoses that is exactly what I did. I was curious to see what was said in those early days when I was too young to understand and whether there was any sign of my other autoimmune conditions throughout my life. Three huge files of PDF documents came through a secure drive on email and I spent a couple of nights reading through them, from the beginning all the way up to the present day.

Looking back through my hospital records, I feel sorry for teenage Sam. The follow-up letters from appointments all spend a needlessly long time talking about how 'Samantha has put on some weight', 'Samantha is eating low carb to try and lose weight', 'Samantha has been eating chocolate'. Every single appointment entry had an unnecessary reference to my weight. So what if I had eaten chocolate? Chocolate is my vice; I could eat it all day every day, but I do not because I carry the burden of diabetes everywhere with me. I do not need to be restrictive with chocolate; I need to make sure I prepare and manage my blood sugar effectively around me eating chocolate.

In the early 2000s TV was full of celebrities promoting a very unattainable size 0. Teenage girls could not escape from the constant 'skinny' expectation. I never had an overweight BMI, I have never been overweight and yet, as viewers of these programmes, my friend and I would compare ourselves to those we saw on screen. We did not have an appreciation that these celebs had private chefs, personal trainers and stylists all working in the background to create this image we were all presented with.

As a fourteen-year-old who was nowhere near overweight, I remember my friends following the 'Special K' diet where they would eat two bowls of cereal a day and one small, low-calorie meal for weeks on end. If you have ever actually weighed out a 30g portion of cereal you will know it hardly touches the sides of a bowl, so you will appreciate how hungry they must have been.

Everyone knew somebody who was following the Atkins diet, Slimming World or Weight Watchers with a view to becoming their smallest self because that was what society expected. When I reached my early 20s, I started to do some more specific reading around low-carb diets for those with type one diabetes. It made sense – less carbs, less insulin, less weight gain. I trialled it, opting for more veggies, less carbs. I would turn down bread whenever it was offered to me. I would sit and watch other people eating jacket potatoes, tummy rumbling whilst I took out my pre-packed lunch of ham slices and hard-boiled eggs. I lost two and half stone of weight that I had carried throughout my university years. I felt better in myself, my clothes were looser, but I was tired. I craved roast potatoes, crisps and chips.

I still follow a relatively 'low-carb' diet but nowhere near the realms of keto. I generally feel better when I can control my blood sugars a bit tighter and for me that means removing the complexity of trying to calculate insulin doses for pasta and bread.

It is really sad to think that diet culture still consumes society almost a quarter of a century later. Some people truly live their life obsessing about food intake, and not for a medical reason but because they think people will feel less of them for looking a certain way. I hate the fact that every time I am presented with a plate of food, the mathematical equations start ticking over in my head and I automatically default to 'well the potatoes will be two units, the vegetables are OK but that's a big bit of chicken so I will probably need to split dose for that amount of protein'. However, what I hate more is that some people feel they have no choice but to eat less to become the skinniest version of themselves because that's what people expect, when really society needs to look at what they can add to their diets – more fruit, more vegetables, more fibre – to make them feel their best self.

One day at school a classmate actually came up to me and said, 'We've been talking about it, Samantha, and you've got a nice figure: you're not the skinniest but you're not the biggest either'. What a weird thing to say to someone! But unfortunately, we do live in a society consumed by the way people look. There is so much more to life than forever dieting, worrying about clothes sizes and comparing the way you look to everyone else around you.

There seems to be a shift happening in society now whereby people feel able to express exactly who they are regardless of what people think. There is a newfound confidence in younger generations that means they will say it how it is and whole heartedly stand up for what they believe in, even in the face of objection. Though unfortunately, there is still a societal expectation to never age, never put on weight and never expect too much. Social media still remains flooded with 'follow my 28-day standing ab workout and drop two stone by Christmas' type of content, which is not healthy for any of us.

The crux of it is – did we ever see our grandparents or great grandparents sit in front of a screen for eight hours a day, obsessing over their protein intake and hitting the gym six times a week? No. They worked jobs that kept their brain active whilst also moving, they ate home-cooked meals at a table socialising with their family, and they spent time enjoying the small things, walking, dancing and keeping the garden looking nice. Somewhere along the road, the human race has prioritised long hours at work, needing as much money in the bank as possible and barely leaving the sofa because of TV binges and social media doom-scrolling on mobile phones. For me, healthy living is all about getting back to the basics. Put your phone down. Eat food where you can understand the ingredient list. Get outside and move in whatever way you can.

My love of food remains strong to this day, and I hope it always is. When I moved into my first house and had my own kitchen, I started experimenting with baking and cooking more. My nan had unfortunately passed away by then, but I took what she taught with me and ran. I would make family and friends birthday cakes, bread, cookies and anything I saw online that I fancied trying to do.

I would spend hours in the kitchen cooking up creations, taking sugar out, using fruit as a natural sweetener instead. I would find ways to fill cakes that did not rely on vast amount of buttercream. When it came to biscuits, I would try and adapt recipes using three types of sugar to just requiring sweetener to see whether it still worked.

My favourite thing to do is hosting a dinner party. Over the years, I have created three-course set menus, put together a pizza party and even turned my kitchen island into a cheese and meat grazing table. I love the creativity that I find when preparing and making food. I always said I wanted to be a solicitor because of the use of words and how one simple word interpreted in the wrong way can lead to a completely different judicial decision. Food is a way of bringing people from different backgrounds and walks of life together to experience unified enjoyment through a common thread. Food is so diverse, so adaptable and something which can bring such joy to so many.

Food is how I express my love for people. There is something so fulfilling about creating something from scratch and watching others enjoy it.

It was not until my mid-20s that I really found exercise. Nowadays most people will go for a run to burn off the takeaway they had the night before or because they had a cake in the staffroom at lunchtime. Sadly, this has what has been drilled into the millennial generation. I decided to run because I could raise awareness by doing it for a charity. I hate running, but it gave me the discipline to keep going.

Many things change as you grow up, and whilst my love for exercise remains, the type and frequency has shifted. I now prioritise my weight training, completing 20-minute YouTube workouts followed by a 10-minute cardio video, rather than going for an hour long run. When my body feels tense or tight, I do yoga. I run when I want to and walk whenever I can. The unswerving promise to myself is to look after my body.

Sometimes that means taking a rest day and only doing 4,000 steps – balance is key.

I generally have a very calm demeanour, but one thing that really triggers me is seeing normal, fully functional, healthy people being conned into buying medical devices or supplements for someone else's financial gain. It has absolutely nothing to do with improving or supporting their health.

The 'blood sugar trend' is something everyone seems to have jumped on board with, gaining real traction in the last year. I read an article in 2024 where scientists questioned this idea ('Doctors question science behind blood sugar diet trend', March 2024, BBC News). Companies were insisting that everyone should wear a continuous glucose monitor (CGM) to understand their blood sugar trends and 'take ownership of their health' or weight loss. This trend targets innocent individuals, particularly those who are health conscious or desperate for answers, encouraging them to spend their money on a blood sugar monitoring device with astronomical fees.

If you have a fully functioning pancreas, you do not need to worry about blood sugar rises after eating food: it is entirely normal. The marketing tactics of using celebrity influencers and scaremongering people into believing the only way to live a healthy life is by paying £200+ for a CGM is complete nonsense.

As a type one diabetic, trust me when I say you do not want to wear one of these devices when you do not need to. It consumes your mind with how your blood sugars are trending and for those of us without a choice, we have to BE THE PANCREAS, whereas those with a fully functioning pancreas can trust their body to do what it needs to do. We diabetics can't rely on our body to do that for us.

Diabetics have to analyse the data presented from a CGM and inject insulin into our bodies based on food, exercise, changes to routine, stress, illness, along with any changes in blood sugar readings. Type one diabetes is not a choice and it is not caused by eating too much sugar; it is an autoimmune disease without a cure.

Sadly, disordered eating is very common within the diabetic community. Demonising food is not the way to live a healthy or happy life. We live in a society which will brand food pumped full of who knows how many additives and preservatives as 'good' in an effort to sell 'high protein', whereas 'bad' food includes bread – which you can make from three simple whole ingredients: flour, water and yeast – no nasties. Bonkers. Ultimately, all food is energy for the body, that is its purpose. Some is simply more nutritious than others and 'diets' often do not work as they are not lifestyle changes: they are quick fixes by means of a short-term calorie deficit through various forms.

We all know which food makes us feel good and which makes us feel crappy, without the added unnecessary complication of 24/7 blood glucose monitoring.

Chapter Five:
Insulin Pump vs MDI

In July 2019 I had a real shock when I secured a charity place in the London Marathon to raise money for Diabetes UK. I had a flashback to the young Sam sat on the end of the hospital bed watching the competitors days after being diagnosed as diabetic. I remember getting the call in the carpark at work on a really hot day and being so excited to get home and tell my husband. Everyone thought I was totally mad, but I grabbed the challenge by the throat and literally ran with it. I was out training three times a week from that very day, increasing my long runs by a mile a week.

I am in no way a natural runner, so it was quite a shock to the system when I realised just how much training was involved. With cancelled weekend plans and endless hours alone, suffering through rain, wind or ice, it's a real hard slog to get marathon ready.

The technology becoming available for diabetics is literally saving lives and making management so much easier. I love my continuous glucose monitor (CGM) and cannot imagine going back to only finger prick testing.

Throughout my teenage years I had discussions around the pump and how it would look, wondering where I would put it when I had a bikini on, what would happen if I got tangled in the tubes.

Pump technology has advanced considerably since those early years. There are now tubeless pumps and closed loop systems which mean a CGM and pump can talk to each other, administering insulin as needed based on the data stored in the technology. The tech is becoming such a useful tool to diabetics, but it can also be a burden.

With all the increased activity, my blood sugars started to become a bit of a rollercoaster and my diabetes team suggested I might like to try an insulin pump. I was nervous, sceptical but willing to give it a go. I was scheduled a half hour appointment with the Diabetes Nurse to set me up. We sat and went through my recent blood sugar readings, carb ratios and insulin doses. Some fancy maths resulted in a set rate which would be delivered to me via the pump all day, every day. I was shown how to program in carbohydrate intake to calculate insulin dose for food and how to suspend insulin delivery if I was exercising. It felt like going back to the day of diagnosis, with the orange, and learning all over again.

Taking diabetes from 'an invisible' to 'a visible' condition hit me a bit harder than I expected. The pump was chunky and easy to knock. It stuck out through clothing and looked odd under jeans.

One morning in August I woke up feeling really 'off', sick, dizzy, lethargic. I tested my levels to find they were

27 mmol (five times above what they should be) and issued a correction dose with my pump. I dragged myself to the shower and had to get out quick to be sick. I came out of the bathroom and sat on the bed. 'Are you OK?' my husband asked. 'Definitely not,' I replied. I measured my blood sugars again and they were still dangerously high. I looked at my pump. I had never felt so ill since my diagnosis.

I decided to take the pump off and give myself an injection of insulin. I examined the device to try and work out what, if anything, was wrong. The cannula to the pump was completely bent and I had not had any insulin all night. It terrified me thinking of what could have happened. I might never have woken up!

These things happen, I know that, but when it literally comes to life or death, and it's your own potential death, it hits differently. I decided at that very moment that the insulin pump was not for me and immediately switched back to injections.

This is not intended to terrify anyone looking to try the pump, for many it works a dream and their blood sugar control is so much better. I would wholeheartedly encourage people to TRY it. After all, if you don't like it, you can always switch back.

MDI stands for 'multiple daily injections'. When I was first diagnosed, I started on two injections a day (one in the morning, one after my tea in the evening). Fast forward to now and I take at least four injections plus any top-ups I need to bring my blood sugar levels down throughout the day. There is no one-size-fits-all for how many injections a diabetic needs in a day (as it depends on so many extenuating circumstances), so it is for everyone individually to find their own rhythm.

Injections have to be given into a muscly area, like your thighs, buttocks, or the tops of your arms. They can lead to some bruising, as you would expect from a normal injection, but they fade after a couple of days. A lot of people ask whether they hurt. The truth is yes, sometimes they do – but thankfully most of the time they don't.

Administering an injection can attract more attention than simply taking out a phone or pump controller. Injections require you to expose your injection site and crank up the dial on your pen. A few times, particularly in work situations, I have been told, 'I could never inject myself. I would rather die!'. For me personally, this is the most ridiculous thing anyone can ever say. Do people really think diabetics want to inject themselves? Is it something we willingly signed up for? Absolutely not. The insensitivity of others is something that can really wear a diabetic down, particular after a number of years with the disease. We do not want sympathy, we certainly do not expect you to understand, but please have a little bit of sensitivity and read the room before you say something stupid.

Over the past couple of years, through Brexit, Covid lockdowns and various political matters around the world, there has been a shortage of medical supplies. I have heard of diabetics having to ration their insulin dosage so they do not run out. I personally have had to switch back to fingerprick blood testing because CGMs were out of stock for months. It is terrifying to think that if anything rocks the supply of prescriptions or medication to the degree that diabetics cannot get their insulin then they will not survive.

At my last clinic appointment, the pump was mentioned again. I think it will be a reoccurring point of discussion for me moving forward and that's OK. I am grateful that the option of a pump is on the table and, when I am ready, I will be able to give it another try. One consultant once asked me what my fear of the pump was. I explained that it was the thought of 'not waking up in the morning, the pump killing me'. The response I got was:

'Well, you could die from a hypo in your sleep too, so what's the difference?'

Remember what I said earlier about saying something stupid?

The big challenge for me now personally is to learn to trust the technology. I need to put my faith in the medical devices, trusting that they will keep me alive, and get over the fear of losing that little bit of control. With injections, I can see if the insulin is cloudy. I know that if I twist the dial to 7, I should get 7 units. With a pump I plug in the numbers and, based on the data, it does its thing. It acts as a pancreas based on what numbers I have set up in the background. In all honesty, that scares me a bit and I need to trust the tech and also have a bit more faith in myself that I can make the change.

Perhaps it was not the right time for me. Perhaps running the marathon was enough strain on my body without trying to change my insulin routine of 18 years. I do not know. What I do know is that everyone's diabetes management is different and you have to do what is right for YOU!

Diabetes is a lifelong lesson and you need to be comfortable (and having fun!) whilst you are learning!

Chapter Six: POI

I went to a girls' grammar high school so many of my early teenage years were spent listening to people talk about how their bodies were changing and their boyfriend dramas. I was tall and slender throughout high school. I had no boobs, no shape and very little interest in boys. Instead, my mind was taken up by a lot of diabetes decisions, appointments and trying to do well at school.

I was desperate to develop boobs like the rest of my friends. Everyone was starting to wear low cut tops and go up a dress size to cater for the big busts they all seemed to get in year 9. I was still completely flat. For my 16th birthday, my aunt got me a birthday card which was a 'spell for bigger boobs' that came with star confetti. We all laughed and joked, and I even chanted the spell in the hope that I would wake up with the DD's I had always dreamt of having.

It was when my 16th birthday came and passed without any sign of periods making an appearance that Mum mentioned it at a routine diabetes clinic appointment. Nobody seemed that concerned at first: the doctors asked the usual questions about family history and explained diabetes could be playing a part given the age I was diagnosed. I was sent for blood tests and then had the normal process of waiting for results. Neither Mum nor I really thought much of it, given nobody seemed that concerned.

Over the course of the next couple of appointments the diabetes team took a little more interest in my puberty development. I was examined on several occasions to see whether 'things were progressing'.

One appointment Mum and I often laugh about is when the Diabetes Consultant asked if it would be OK if the student sat in to listen to my appointment. We went about the usual blood sugar review / insulin dose adjustment conversation before the 'Do you mind if we examine your development?' question came along. I looked at the young male student in the corner and replied, 'Well, I'm sorry but I have got a thong on!' Everyone burst out laughing and it thankfully lightened the mood, as well as taking the embarrassment away from me and the poor student.

Thankfully, not many teens have to worry about puberty examinations, it just happens for them. Many women face a natural apprehension of cervical smear tests as it will be the first time they have had to expose themselves in front of medical professionals. Sadly, that dignity for me was taken in those early years. I have had so many doctors, nurses, students look at all different parts of me over the course of the past 20 years, smear tests were just another string to the bow.

When I hit the age of 17, the results of some blood tests came back and I was sent for an internal CT scan. Without going into too much detail, which I am pretty sure nobody would want to hear, it was a horrific experience. I joke about it now, but no teenage girl should have to go through that. The scan results were where it was confirmed I had one tiny ovary and no eggs or 'follicles' within it. 'You have primary ovarian failure' (as it was then called…) didn't really register with me.

Primary ovarian failure has been relabelled 'primary ovarian insufficiency' or 'POI' in recent years. The removal of the word failure suggests that it's not something the patient has done wrong – it's not as a result of any action taken by the individual but rather it is because the body is lacking in something. Failure is a funny word, but I personally am not sure insufficiency is much better. The technical definition of POI is a woman's ovaries stopping working before the age of 40. In my case my ovaries stopped working at least twenty-seven years before they were supposed to. Nobody knows why it happens as there is no definitive cause of the condition and there is still hardly any information around POI at all.

Following my diagnosis with POI at the age of 17, I graciously went along to an infertility clinic with my mum. We sat in the waiting room surrounded by couples who looked lost. The atmosphere was cold, not loving or excited, but consumed with a cloud of bitterness, resentment and fear. I sat wondering why I was there, thinking that I didn't want children yet so what was the point of this exercise? I remember Mum looked quite anxious, but we sat chatting away whilst those around us remained in icy silence. We watched countless men go in through a door with little cups, an endless line of them in and out.

The appointment was brief and direct. We met with a male consultant in his 50s, someone that I could not relate to at all. I was told I would not be able to conceive a child naturally as part of the usual course of life. He went on to say I would need an egg donor if I ever wanted to have children. Back then, he said that as I had been diagnosed as infertile I would be entitled to receive one free round of IVF. I remember the tone of his voice making me think, 'am I supposed to be grateful?' His quick caveat on the back of his statement was that the freebie was only valid up until I was 37 (after that I would be considered too high risk so there would be a charge).

The final point he made was that I would need to be placed on medication to ensure my womb was fit to carry a child in the future and I was sent on my merry way. I cannot remember asking any questions at all. I think Mum asked a few but I could not relate to having children at the age of 17. They were not on my radar. I wanted to go to uni, travel, have fun and think about being an adult when I was one. Not as a child myself. I had no long-term boyfriend (no boyfriend at all, in fact!) so the thought of having to think about 'adult' things at such a young age must have been pretty overwhelming.

After that appointment, I again took it in my stride. I joked about how I would be able to keep my abs and went on with life as usual.

I hardly gave the POI diagnosis any thought at all until I grew older. I went to university and got my dream degree. I then spent the next few years making sure I qualified in the profession I had always dreamt I would. I got married, bought a house, got a dog.

In fact, it was not until my early 30s, when I found social media consumed by 'perimenopause' and 'menopause' awareness campaigns. We are constantly shown stories of celebrities on their 'fertility journey', choosing to freeze eggs or have their tenth child because 'they still have it at 45'. When I sat in that freezing cold fertility clinic there was no talk of trying to extract any eggs I did have and freezing them. There was no talk about what I could do to try and understand what 'normal hormones' were for me. There was absolutely no mention at all of how to manage this condition in later life (i.e. not as a teenager just trying to get through two years of sixth form).

Over the next few years, I would be called to the doctors' for an 'annual pill check'. I had been prescribed a contraceptive mini pill with combined progesterone and oestrogen to make sure that, if I decided to have IVF, my womb would be in a state to potentially carry a child. At each and every appointment from the age of 17, without fail, the first question I would be asked was: 'is there any chance you could be pregnant?' It used to infuriate me. Why would it not be tagged at the top of the doctor's screen that I was not on this pill because I was a rampant teenager looking for a good time but because I had a crushing diagnosis that meant I was on this road for 'treatment'. I would snap back 'if you read my notes, you will see I have primary ovarian failure, so fat chance of being pregnant'. The look back would always be one of terror, but they should have known better.

It triggered a number of questions in my head as to whether I would ever experience menopause or whether I had experienced menopause already? Should I have seen warning signs at 16 that something wasn't right? Hot flushes? Mood changes? Should I have asked about not starting my period sooner? Instead of doing spells to make my boobs grow, should I have raised my concerns with the doctors?

I never once considered myself to have gone through menopause. Menopause has this awful connotation of an old woman drying up and having hot sweats. That had never been me. I had not noticed any signs of menopause at all. Thankfully, the narrative on menopause seems to be shifting: many companies now even have menopause policies and awareness campaigns to advocate for all the different symptoms that come along with it. That being said, it makes me uncomfortable to think I am in my early 30s and have already been through menopause. 'Wait 'til you get to my age' hits a little differently when you know you are not going to go through what they are because your body decided that was not the way things were going to pan out for you.

I decided to take the bull by the horns and reach out to a specialist on Instagram. She so kindly pointed me to a local specialist and gave me a name to reach out to. Her message clearly said, 'You should be under a specialist. You have 'polyendocrine syndrome'.' Of course I defaulted to Google, checking as to what polyendocrine syndrome was and how it could affect me moving forward. The thing that really annoyed me was that in over 20 years as a diabetic, and now with other autoimmune conditions raising their ugly head, this was the first time I had ever heard that term.

I decided to spend the money and get a private appointment with the recommended specialist. I thought at length about whether I could justify the money. I wanted to be very clear with myself what I wanted to achieve from the appointment. I was keen to understand what was going on with my body – was this my fault? Was this unfortunate string of diagnoses preventable? Should I be doing yoga or eating more spinach?

The second and probably most important question for me was to determine whether there was anything I could do myself to ensure I was in control going forward. If I was in the depths of menopause, should I be eating pumpkin seeds for extra magnesium at breakfast? Was there anything left in my control that meant I could stop, prevent or fix all these autoimmune issues?

In those forty-five minutes I learned more about hormones than anyone had ever taken the time to explain to me before. The consultant took the time to listen to my checklist of questions I had written in my notebook. They listened to me run through my medical history and all the challenges I had faced over the years.

I got the clarity I so desperately wanted. It was confirmed that there was simply nothing more I could add to or remove from my already healthy lifestyle to have prevented POI from happening was reassuring.

The sad part was that the condition is something which is just the same as diabetes: incurable, lifelong and totally life changing.

The appointment made me feel more settled in my skin than I had done for a long time. I held a resentment for my body which I could not shake off and I think, in hindsight, it was because I felt we were fighting against each other.

A letter was sent to my GP suggesting that my hormone treatment should be changed to hormone replacement therapy (HRT) rather than the combined contraceptive pill I had been taking for fifteen years without review, no questions asked.

I felt nervous changing my medication as I did not know what to expect. I started the HRT a couple of months ago and find myself now wondering if I feel any different, which I do not think I do, or whether I feel 'more balanced'. No idea.

I am childless and happy. There is no appeal to me in going on the journey to have a child, personally. There are a lot of women out there desperate to be mothers and there is nowhere near enough awareness or support for those diagnosed with POI.

Chapter Seven: Coeliac Disease

'Google it'. That was the advice I received from the nurse at the hospital when I received my coeliac diagnosis and I asked what it meant. I felt like I had been punched in the stomach for the third time in a hospital – part of the initiation to join a club nobody would want to be in: a club for people with three different autoimmune diseases.

Coeliac disease is an autoimmune condition where someone's immune system attacks their small intestine in response to gluten, which is found in wheat, barley and rye. Common symptoms of coeliac disease include stomach bloating, vomiting and diarrhoea. Some lesser-known effects of the condition are infertility, rashes and numbness. I had no symptoms at all, absolutely nothing.

An endoscopy is not a pleasant experience. You are conscious whilst a tube is pushed down your throat and a biopsy of your gut is taken.

Over my teenage years and early 20s the routine blood tests they do as part of the annual diabetic review kept coming back above normal. The results would go up and down with no obvious correlation as to why. The diabetes consultants were insistent that more tests should be done to find out whether or not I had coeliac disease. As a result, over the course of 18 years, I underwent four intrusive endoscopies for them all to come back 'inconclusive'. My mum and I look back and laugh at the experiences we had, one time we went to the hospital for an endoscopy the day before we flew out on holiday, with no idea what an endoscopy entailed. Another time, I had the endoscopy on my birthday, so we went out for mashed potatoes as a celebratory lunch.

My favourite endoscopy (how sad that I have a favourite?!) was number three of five. I was apprehensive of the appointment knowing what was coming and obviously subconsciously decided to be difficult. The doctor told my mum 'we've given her enough sedative to knock out a baby elephant and her eyes are still open'. We laughed so much when I came round, true Sam fashion.

At a diabetes clinic appointment in summer 2023 the consultant mentioned that my blood test results showed a higher level than they would like on one of my results and that this could be coeliac disease. They advised it would be best if I underwent an endoscopy.

I sat in the chair, looking at a consultant I had met a couple of times previously and their student, and said clearly, 'I don't want one. Can I not just follow a gluten free diet and see if the levels improve?'

'You will live a miserable existence if you follow a gluten free diet.'

I reluctantly agreed to have one final endoscopy and made it clear I had absolutely no intention of undergoing the procedure ever again. I should have really known. An appointment came through for six weeks later.

Three weeks before my scheduled endoscopy my husband and I went to Ibiza. I declined burgers and chips, opting for salads to make blood sugar management easier. When we came back to the UK autumn had hit and we started getting the cosy comfort food on the go for dinner. Stew and dumplings, sausage and mash, roast dinners...

The night before my endoscopy we had a steak and onion pie, veg and gravy. It was my last gluten-filled meal, and it was utterly delicious. I can still remember the taste of the flaky pastry and thick gravy.

The next morning, I felt sick at the thought of what was coming.

My husband and I sat in the sweltering waiting room, reading the signs on the wall waiting for me to be called in. One benefit of being diabetic means you can ask to be first on the list for procedures which require you to fast. As the minutes clocked by, I was eventually called through to get changed. My husband asked if he could stay but was told the doctor hadn't arrived yet and could be some time. They would give him a ring when I was ready to be collected. I smiled and assured him it was fine. In reality, I wanted to leave with him.

In the side room, a cannula was inserted into my vein ready for the sedative. The nurse was kind and we put the world to rights, chatting away as she distracted me from what was to come. Dressed in a hospital gown, although this time thankfully I could keep my leggings on, I took a selfie and sent it to my husband to let him know I was OK.

The consultant conducting the procedure asked me whether I'd had an endoscopy before. I went through my history, explaining that I had received four 'inconclusive' results in the past and that I just wanted an answer either way. The consultant asked what symptoms I experienced that had led to me undergoing so many procedures. I explained I had no symptoms at all, not one. 'No problem, Sam, we will take plenty of biopsies and pictures to get you an answer either way.'

Tears streamed down my face as I gagged. The Nurse stroked my cheek.

'Well, Sam, you have got coeliac disease. Look at this!'

I was shown the pictures of my gut and listened as the doctor explained the villi in my intestine should be standing up but mine were totally flat. Damaged from eating gluten. Essentially, this means that my gut was not absorbing nutrients as it should. A lot of those suffering with coeliac disease experience symptoms such as stomach cramps, wind or bloating and that makes total sense from what I saw on the screen. Without nutrients how are we supposed to function properly? Food is energy after all.

The words 'miserable existence' echoed in my ears as soon as the doctor confirmed I had coeliac disease.

I have not been able to shake them out of my mind even now, over a year post diagnosis.

I sat in the recovery wing waiting for the sedative to wear off before they would release me home. I took another selfie, not quite as smiley this time. I thought about the Baileys truffle advent calendar at home that I had bought only the day before. When the nurse came round, I asked, 'The doctor says I've got coeliac disease. What does that mean?'

She replied, 'You need to eat gluten free. Google it.'

Taken aback, the questions kept on coming: 'Gluten free from now? Or when I get the diagnosis come through officially?'

'Now.'

I sat there in disbelief. What had just happened? What did this mean? Is this what chronic illness diagnosis had become, a case of just googling it? There was nothing else to do, so I googled it! That was when I felt the wave of grief return. It took me over as it had in my early diabetes days (although I had not acknowledged it then, reflecting on it far more as a teenager). The sadness of knowing what was and what now had to be.

When my husband picked me up, he walked in smiling. I just looked at him and said 'positive' and the smile disappeared. He looked shell-shocked and confused, an expression I can still clearly remember to this day.

The diagnosis did not hit me for a while. The first food shop was (and continues to be) a real mental struggle. The constant reading of labels for 'contains' or 'may contain', the mixture of emotions as you cross your fingers that your favourite seasonal treat is gluten free only to feel the crushing disappointment or realising that, in your new world, it is off limits. My diagnosis was pretty close to Christmas, which meant I had already started stocking up on goodies. It turned out that I could not eat any of them. I sat with a deep sadness watching others enjoying all of the festive treats I had bought or made, pleased they were having a great time but upset that I had to watch from the sidelines this time.

Within three days of my diagnosis, my husband had ordered me a 'gluten free quick guide' and my best friend had 'Becky Excell's, Gluten Free Christmas' delivered. Those little heartwarming gestures meant everything; it was all going to be OK.

The coeliac diagnosis took me right back to those early diabetes days, with everyone feeling sorry for me and putting on their sad expressions as I explained what coeliac disease meant.

Next up was to go through all the cupboards and read all of the labels. I had two piles: 'gluten' and 'gluten free'. A few store cupboard items surprised me: stock cubes, Daddies brown sauce, Doritos? Beyond the very obvious things that contain gluten, like bread, flour and pasta, there really are a lot of items out there that you would not believe have gluten in. My husband and I agreed we would start to phase out a lot of the 'gluten' pile and keep gluten free alternatives in the cupboard instead where we could.

My best friend and I had a girls' weekend booked a few weeks post diagnosis and needed to find somewhere for dinner. Now I know all coeliacs reading this will relate when I say eating out with this disease is an absolute minefield! We studied the menus of the restaurants nearby to where we were staying and picked Miller & Carter – steak is always a winner in my books. Miller & Carter are to this day one of my favourite restaurants. They have a separate gluten free menu, which almost mirrors the traditional menu, and the staff (from my experience) understand the need to ensure no cross-contamination. Needless to say, the experience that weekend did not reflect the experiences I have had dining out since!

I have been asked 'How serious is your gluten allergy?' and often get told 'Well, we will try and not touch non-gluten free food' by servers.

Next on the list of new experiences with coeliac was an appointment with a dietician. My relationship with food definitely shifted post diagnosis. I spent a lot of time analysing my plate, looking at labels, and I noticed I was starting to obsess a little too much over food. Diabetes and coeliac combined definitely make for an unhappy relationship with your diet. The research around patients suffering with one or both conditions shows an increased likelihood of disordered eating and that is because treatment of both really does orientate around food.

I met with a lovely lady who explained more about the gut not absorbing nutrients and asked what blood tests I had been referred for to see whether I was malnourished in any way. I had not been sent for any, which her blank computer screen confirmed. I explained about my diabetes and how I was driven to live a healthy lifestyle full of a wide variety of foods and lots of exercise. She agreed that there seemingly was nothing more I could do in terms of diet but just to be mindful of cross-contamination in the home. I learned about prescriptions and that, in some areas of the UK, it is possible to request bread and pasta on prescription, given the huge cost of them in the shops. I was sent away with a blood form and told they would be in touch if there was anything more to discuss.

Two days after my blood test, I had a call from the doctors requesting an urgent telephone appointment. My results had shown I was anaemic and needed to take iron tablets for three months to boost my levels. I compliantly took the pills and never heard anything more.

Travelling with coeliac disease can be tricky but one tip for all those newly diagnosed – always be prepared! My first holiday was only six weeks post diagnosis to go and visit Santa in Lapland. I had been looking forward to the trip for over a year and, as soon as I was diagnosed, messaged the travel agent to ask about gluten-free options, as we were half board. The holiday was fantastic and I loved every second, but wow did it put things in perspective about the lack of awareness around gluten free options whilst out and about.

On the aeroplane, there were two gluten free options, a vegan brownie packed full of sugar or a bag of vegetable puffs for babies. Everyone around me was tucking into their ham and cheese panini whilst I chomped on baby crisps.

The second time was on an excursion where pasta was the set menu option for everyone. Two huge pots of cheesy, tomato pasta were steaming in the middle of the table, accompanied by a table of bread and then a salad bar. I was presented with a bowl of cucumber and lettuce - the only gluten free option again.

The key message here is: carry snacks whenever you are out and about. I have no shame now in cracking out my protein bar if a restaurant cannot cater for me. Never trust TripAdvisor reviews either: I have been caught out a couple of times by a 'fantastic gluten free choices' or 'catered for my gluten intolerance' review only to find that truth was quite the opposite. Remember – it's a them problem, not a you problem!

One thing I do now if I am invited out to eat is to check ahead. Check all the menus before you agree to go anywhere and make sure they can cater for your needs to a degree you personally feel comfortable with. if they look confused when you ask if their gluten free chips are cooked in a separate fryer, then it's a no go for me!

Last year, my husband and I went to the Caribbean on holiday. After landing quite late at night, we were hungry and tired and went to the first restaurant we could find on site. It was a British pub themed restaurant, with all the usual classics we know and love. I asked which items on the menu were gluten free and was told 'everything's gluten free here'. My husband took great delight in asking if that included the 'beer battered fish and chips' to which the response was 'yes of course, all gluten free'. I opted for a steak and salad just to be safe!

The first Christmas as a coeliac is a total blur. Christmas is my absolute favourite time of year. The lights, the cheer, the fizz and the food. Spending a few days away from work with those you love, doing what you want when you want, is just the best feeling in the world.

We were hosting Christmas dinner (which we love to do) and I was insistent everyone else would have their usual gluten-filled stuffing, pigs in blankets and gravy. I would make my dinner completely separate from everyone else's to make sure only I noticed a difference. I agonised over keeping things separate. There were trays all over the kitchen worktops and endless hand washing. I even had pre-empted the chaos and bought myself disposable gloves, which came on and off throughout the Christmas prep. I felt a huge sense of disappointment that I have never had on Christmas before as I sat down at the table and looked at the food in front of me. On reflection, there was literally almost nothing different. The texture of the shop-bought gluten free stuffing was a little off. I think that one hurt because I decided this year would be the one I would make everyone else homemade stuffing with sausagemeat, lemon and thyme and they all raved about how 'it was the best stuffing they had ever tasted'.

Lesson learnt: buy gluten free sausagemeat next year. I ate my dinner and it was OK, but I had a big cloud over me as I felt like I had missed out. Not this year!

Time flew by and BBQ season quickly followed. My husband invited my best friend and her family round for the first BBQ of the year and I panicked. 'How do we make this gluten free and avoid cross-contamination?', 'The kids don't want gluten free sausages, so what can I feed them?' and so many other questions all raced through my mind.

Next thing I knew, there was my best friend's husband wheeling round his BBQ to make sure nobody else's food was anywhere near mine. The BBQ was fantastic, the company, the food, but when everyone left and I got into bed, I burst into tears. I could not believe how much extra effort people went to so they could make sure I was safe. I always hated the feeling of being awkward and I still do.

More recently, we spent a weekend down London with our best friends. We went for a drink in a hotel bar but it was a couple of hours until our booked evening meal. I took a look at the menu and asked whether the nachos were gluten free. 'No,' the bartender snapped back. I continued looking and asked, 'What about your chips? Are they gluten free?' After a slight pause they laughed and said, 'Duh they are potatoes'. I felt a wave of rage consume me but smiled sweetly. 'Oh, I know they are potatoes, but do you use a separate fryer or are you frying your battered fish in the same oil? Do you have any way to not cross-contaminate food as I am coeliac'

Well, I think they got the hint. 'Let me talk to the chef'. I had absolutely no intention of eating any of the food they were going to suggest was gluten free. The staff member came over with two bags, one popcorn, one crisps. They showed me the bag of popcorn, apologised and said as it was gluten free. They would be happy to provide this alongside our drinks. The crisps were not gluten free, but I did smile as they came out in a separate bowl and placed completely the other end of the table away from me!

I have found that since being diagnosed as coeliac, dinner invitations have dwindled. I completely understand: people are terrified of contaminating me and that's OK. I love hosting and I am happy to do so. Those that go out of their way to host you for food and make sure everything they prepare is gluten free, so there is no chance of cross-contamination, don't go unnoticed and it genuinely makes me feel so much more included in things when I do not have to be the awkward one asking 'is this gluten free?' as I add things to my plate.

The summer continued and we were invited to my husband's work colleague's house for a BBQ. I didn't know him particularly well so politely declined and stayed home. As someone who has always loved hosting and being sociable it hit me like a ton of bricks that this was my life now. I either had to suck it up and be the 'awkward one' at gatherings or I would miss out on everything.

Since being diagnosed as a silent coeliac on top of type one diabetes, I have felt more than ever before just how much unnatural focus has to be put onto food choices.

Please do not follow the crowd and feel peer pressured into things that do not sit right with you. Trust your body and enjoy the small things; if you personally do not feel comfortable eating at an establishment, you are not obligated to do so. Be selfish – your health always comes first.

Chapter Eight: Live Your Dreams

Any medical diagnosis can have a negative effect on your attitude. Throw in the fact that you are responsible for keeping yourself alive and your dreams and ambitions can become a little overwhelming. I have always had big plans in life and been very much a 'glass half full' kind of woman, certainly over the past ten years or so.

One of my favourite sayings from an old boss was 'control the controllables'. When you attribute this to life, it becomes a hell of a lot easier! I often find myself reflecting on diabetes decisions, or even work challenges, with the question, 'what can I control here?' Funnily enough, the answer usually makes the next step so much easier to navigate.

From the age of seven, I used to tell everyone I was going to be a solicitor and you know what? Despite the challenges thrown my way, I did it! No part of it was easy, and it took me a fair few years to get there, but I did it and that gives me such great satisfaction to know diabetes did not stop me.

I remember my mum's face back in July 2019 when I told her I was going to run the London Marathon.

She looked scared and anxious, but I reassured her I'd got this and was willing to put in the work to raise the money for Diabetes UK.

I spent the next two years training (thanks Covid!) and fighting the rollercoaster of diabetes management to make sure that I was fit enough to finish. 'What finish time are you aiming for?' people would ask. I would have the same response every single time: 'I just want to finish it alive!'

The marathon itself was a real test of mental grit when it came to my diabetes. I decided to drink nothing but water in the weeks leading up to the race, so as to not have anything to look back on and say, 'I wish I had...' My diet was healthy, full of protein and all fuel sources came in the form of homemade energy flapjack full of dried fruit. The morning of the race came and my husband and mum had joined me in London to watch it. We were staying at a gorgeous hotel, and I had laid out all of my kit the night before ready for me to pin on my number. We had to set off early, which meant breakfast needed to be quick and easy. I had taken my own two Weetabix and mixed nuts in a sandwich bag. We had stopped at the Tesco Express the night before to pick up some skimmed milk and I sat in my mum's hotel room dressed like an athlete, eating Weetabix from a mug with a teaspoon. My husband and mum tried to steady my nerves as the enormity of the day ahead started to sink in.

I was dropped off at the start line. This was it. The moment I had been training for for over two years had finally arrived. I tested my blood sugars to see where the adrenalin was taking me. I was sat at 11 mmol, exactly where I wanted to be at the start of the long run. Before I knew it, the time had come and we were off: I was running the London Marathon!

Over the first half of the race I was so excited by the atmosphere and all the people around me. I spotted one runner who had lost both legs and was running on prosthetics. 'An anonymous someone has donated £5,000 to my JustGiving page this morning,' I heard as I jogged past. 'You deserve every penny of that,' I thought. As I hit London Bridge, the spectators in the crowd were electric. I threw my hands in the air and took it all in, the blue sky, the banners waving, the clapping and yelping of those around me. As I hit halfway, I called my husband and mum to let them know I was OK. I could not hear a word they said but what I could see on WhatsApp video was their two cocktail glasses chinking in the Hard Rock Cafe! They are OK, I am OK. 'What a great day this is!' I thought.

I carried on and at mile 21 I started to really flag. I tested my blood sugar, which had crept up to 19mmol from the adrenalin. I decided to take a loo break and walk a little bit to let my body settle. It worked and by mile 23 I was jogging along again. I saw the London Eye in the distance and felt a huge wave of excitement rush through my body. I burst into tears and the tears did not stop flowing for the next three miles. A mixture of relief, joy and – dare I say it – a tinge of sadness over the fact that this mammoth event was almost over all collided meaning I could not hold it together. The final sprint down Pall Mall was indescribable – a moment I will never forget for as long as I live.

On the train home I sat (thankfully!) clutching my medal with a huge smile on my face – once again, diabetes had not won.

Will I run a marathon again? Absolutely not, never again. Would I encourage you to have a go? One hundred percent! Everyone should experience it, and if I can do it, so can you!

My passion for food led me on a very unexpected path to London… I first saw the Instagram post by Fortnum and Mason about the Platinum Pudding competition one day in January when I was scrolling through with a morning coffee. The competition was inviting home bakers from across the UK to submit a recipe and photo of their submission for a pud to be crowned the 'Platinum Pudding' in celebration of the late Queen's seventy years on the throne. I had been to Fortnum and Mason once and instantly loved the shop. It had such elegance but felt 'homely' and the foodhall was every foodie's dream!

I thought about the competition for a while and mentioned it to my mum. I talked her through my plan to make a simple Victoria sponge cake in the shape of a crown. Mum told me how she had read that the late Queen was known for liking a drink of Dubonnet fortified wine and suggested I incorporate it into my recipe. I ordered myself a silicone bundt mould from eBay and waited for it to arrive.

The bundt mould arrived on a wet Saturday, perfect for a bit of baking. I got to work making the jam from scratch for the first time in my life and made the traditional sponge, just as I always had been taught. I whipped up another batch of sponge for my brand-new mould and kept everything crossed that my vision would work. Once the cakes had a chance to cool, I looked at the bundt mould and wondered what was going to happen when I flipped it over. 'This is where it all goes wrong,' I thought. It came out in one piece, with perfect colouration and no breakages – a success!

I began decorating the cake very simply, with fresh berries, vanilla buttercream and my homemade Dubonnet-flavoured jam. I ran up to the nearest Aldi and bought some red, blue and white flowers, staged them around my cake and took photos from all angles. I had three critics for the photos – all voting on which should be submitted – and the one with the most votes won. I set out my recipe and submitted my photo, never thinking anything would come of it.

At the time I posted the photo on my Instagram page and used the hashtags set out in the competition guidance. Friends and family commented and kept asking whenever they saw me, 'What's going on with the Queen's cake then?'

A few weeks later, I had an email to say I had made the final 50 of the competition. I could not believe it! I was so excited but sworn to secrecy. I found out I made the top 5 finalists on my birthday. I was beaming. I could not believe it was happening. I was invited down to the Fortnum & Mason kitchens to bake my cake for celebrity judges.

The entire experience of spending those two days with the Fortnum's chef, front of house team and management is something I will hold dear forever. The team were absolutely phenomenal, so kind and welcoming to us all. To be able to say I have cooked in one of the most prestigious kitchens in London, known for its afternoon teas and being known as the grocer to the royal family, is still surreal. I loved every second of the experience. Meeting the four other fabulous finalists was a joy, and we bonded instantly. We were all amateur home bakers, and none of us ever expected to make the final. We shared in our awe of watching the way the professional chefs read our minds and bought us utensils before we had even asked for them – it was like they knew what was coming ten steps ahead and were always prepared.

The whole experience of creating the 'jubilee bundt' opened so many unexpected doors to foodie events and discussions about the world I am so passionate about. I will be forever grateful to Fortnum & Mason for the opportunity and ongoing support in my mission to raise awareness around living with autoimmune conditions.

There was a point in April 2023 when diabetes did unfortunately win. Off the back of a successful marathon attempt, and all the buzz of being down London for the platinum jubilee pudding competition, I decided I was going to attempt the three peaks challenge to raise more money for charity.

The challenge involves climbing Ben Nevis, Scafell and Snowdon in 24hrs, travelling between the mountains and getting up and down all three within a day. I was fit, I was at the gym four or five times a week, mixing up cardio and weights. In the run up to the challenge, I started doing some incline walks to get my legs ready for what was to come. A couple of my friends and my husband agreed to do the challenge with me. I was so grateful for that. We booked through an organised challenge group so that we did not have to drive or worry about finding transport between the mountains. We just had to show up and climb… she says.

We travelled up to Scotland with Ben Nevis being the first mountain on the list. We stayed in a hotel the night before and met with the other members of our group. I did not anticipate being placed in a group with four early 20-year-old men who were wired the same as mountain goats. The challenge was explained to us, by our guide who was thankfully female and a similar age to me. We would all become very cosy in a minibus together over the next couple of days, eating and sleeping with only two breaks from the travel to make sure the drivers could change over.

On the morning of the challenge, I woke up ready. I felt good, my sugars were a little higher than optimal, but I was happy with them knowing what was to come. The hotel had put on breakfast early and I stuck to my usual fruit and yoghurt. I tested my blood sugars a couple of times before we started our ascent.

As we started to climb, I realised I had hugely underestimated what was involved. The terrain was rocky, the temperature kept changing and it was packed with other people. I tested my sugars a couple of times before my CGM lost connection due to the cold weather. I had to resort to fingerprick blood testing, which in itself was hard as I had to keep stopping, getting the kit out, warming up my hands and waiting for the countdown to give me a result. My sugars were now high, probably due to the adrenalin, so I took a small injection to try and bring them down a little. The mountain goats were off, miles ahead, whilst my husband continued to stick close by to keep a check on me. As we got three quarters of the way up, different members of the group were taking it in turns to check on me and make sure I was doing OK.

The guide called us all together to explain the top of Ben Nevis had around 6 feet of snow on it and we would need to assess conditions once we got a bit closer. It was shortly after this that my energy completely depleted. Another blood test and my levels were low. I got a snack out of my backpack and tried to keep up the pace so as not to slow the rest of the group down. When I say the top of the mountain was snowy, imagine Finland on Christmas week. It was magical to look at, absolutely horrific to try and trudge through when your blood sugar levels have plummeted.

Everyone else in the group was layering up, getting ready to brave the cold. I was so delirious I wore just a jumper and carried my coat. My hypo continued for half of the descent so I do not recall a lot of it, but the group guide kept checking to make sure I was OK and giving me a time status update. When we neared the bottom and I could almost see the minibus, my husband made me check my sugars again as I was walking with my back almost parallel to the floor. My sugars were still in my brand-new walking boots, so more snacks were pulled out and eaten. As I boarded the minibus, everyone else who had finished over half an hour earlier said what a good job I had done and that I should be proud.

The drive from Ben Nevis to Scafell involved a stop at a motorway services. The group guide came over for a quiet word and explained to me she was concerned about me doing the next mountain in the dark, given what I had experienced with my blood sugars in the daylight. She also explained how quickly the group needed to get up and down the mountain to meet the twenty-four hour target, politely suggesting I would need to move more quickly and keep up with the rest to make the time.

I burst into tears at the thought of not completing the challenge. We all had a pasty and got back on the stinking bus.

When we reached Scafell, I felt horrendous. I was tired, cold and felt very sick from the low blood sugar chasing with snacks. It was pitch black and the terrain was very unstable. There was no path like we had at Ben Nevis. The route we needed to take was steep and rocky. I lasted about 20 minutes before the guide said I was too slow and the rest would be put in danger if I continued as she would need to be able to watch them and me, which was impossible. I burst into tears. This was it. The first time diabetes had beat me in 22 years. I felt awful, defeated, a letdown. I reluctantly turned back and my husband joined me, supporting me with kind words the whole way down.

As we neared the car park where the bus was waiting for us, we saw two more headlights coming our way. Our two friends had also turned back saying the terrain was too dangerous and, if they continued, they would need to be slower, holding the others back. The four of us got back on the stinky bus, threw blankets over our heads and tried to get a couple of hours sleep.

The goats were on track for achieving their time on Snowdon so we agreed our group would let them carry on ensuring that they could hit the twenty-four hour target. A couple of us had a trundle up the path at our own pace and turned back round when we had enough.

That challenge was a defining moment for me. In the darkness on Scafell I realised I was not invincible and that some things in life were going to be that little bit harder for me.

I know it is not fair that you, me or one of your friends or family have been diagnosed with these conditions, but do you know what? It is not going to change! Make the most of it and do not let these autoimmune diseases win.

Life passes by so quickly, wallowing in self-pity at the life you once knew gets you nowhere. Do not get me wrong, there are days I think 'sod it, I am done with all this' and I give myself a good talking to, have one of my husband's home roasted coffees, pick myself up and go for a walk. There is no choice when it comes to living with an autoimmune condition, but there is control.

We all control the course of our life (in terms of the controllables) so grab it and run! Live your best life!

Favourite Recipes

I found my love for cooking and baking at a young age. Now I have some life experience of living with autoimmune conditions, I hope others enjoy my recipes and find their love of food once again!

Please note: these recipes have not been tested in kitchens or staged by food stylists – these are my own homemade goodies and recipes that I have been using over the years.

To work out the carb count for these recipes, so you can calculate your insulin dose, you will need to do some maths! I have purposefully not included the carb count as I know serving sizes (and appetites!) vary person-to-person.

To calculate the approximate carbs of these home-baked goodies:

1. Add the carbs from each of your ingredients to get a 'total carbs' and divide this by the weight of the finished product. This gives you the approximate carb count for 1g.
2. Weigh your portion and then multiply it by the 1g figure.

GLUTEN FREE CHEESE & ONION FOCACCIA

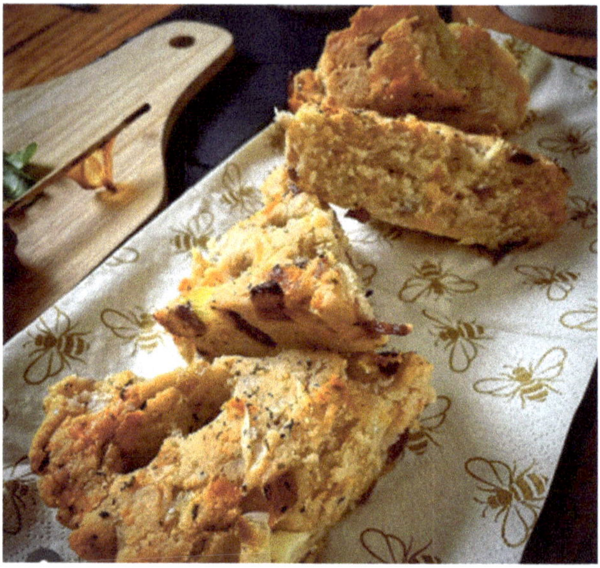

Ingredients

300g gluten free plain flour
200g almond flour
1tsp xanthum gum
14g gluten free yeast
60ml olive oil
100ml water
1 x red onion
Cheese of your choice
Sea salt

1. Preheat your oven to 200 degrees.
2. Add both flours, yeast, xanthum gum and oil to a bowl.
3. Slowly add the water until the dough forms and comes away from the sides of the bowl.
4. Gently knead the dough for a couple of minutes and return to the bowl. Leave in a warm place for 45mins.
5. Meanwhile, fry your onion and grate your cheese.
6. Add the onion and cheese to your dough and place in your tray, loaf tin or form rolls as desired.
7. Leave for 60mins.
8. Press your fingers into the top of the dough to form the focaccia dips, sprinkle with sea salt and a drizzle of olive oil and some more cheese as desired.
9. Cook for 40mins and serve warm.

GLUTEN FREE BEEF AND MUSHROOM PIE

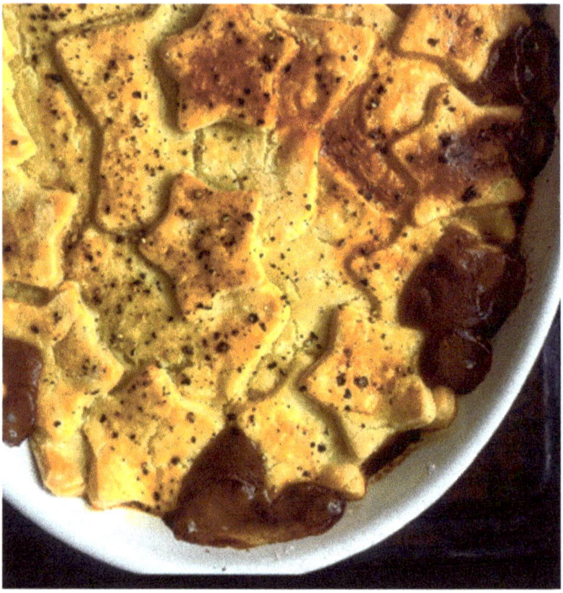

Ingredients

Gluten free shortcrust pastry
250g stewing beef
A generous handful of mushrooms
50g gluten free plain flour
2 x onions
2 x beef stock cubes dissolved in 600ml of water
2tbsp tomato puree
Salt and Pepper
1 x egg and milk for egg washing the pastry

1. Heat a little olive oil in a saucepan and add the beef.
2. Add the flour and fry until the meat turns brown.
3. Add all the mushrooms, beef stock, puree, salt and pepper to the pan.
4. Place the lid on your saucepan and leave to simmer on low heat for 2.5 hours.
5. Place your pie filling in a casserole dish and top with your pastry (you can make your own, buy ready-made and completely style the top of your pie as you wish!).
6. Whisk your egg with a little milk with a fork and brush the mix on top your pie.
7. Cook in the oven for 40mins until golden brown and piping hot.

GLUTEN FREE CHILLI CHEESE CHICKEN NUGGETS

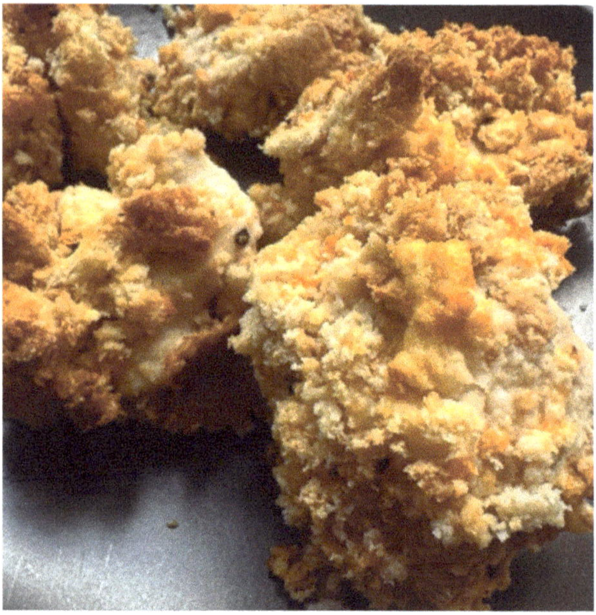

Ingredients

2 x chicken breasts
4 x slices gluten free bread
5tbsp gluten free flour
2 x eggs
Grated chilli cheese
Salt and pepper

1. Preheat your oven to 180 degrees.
2. Use your fingers to make breadcrumbs from the slices of bread and spread them onto a dinner plate.
3. Use a fork to whisk your eggs in a separate bowl and place your flour spread out on a side plate.
4. Add your grated cheese, salt and pepper to the plate of breadcrumbs.
5. Dip your chicken chunk in flour, then egg, then into the breadcrumbs.
6. Place on a lined baking tray and bake for 30mins until golden brown and cooked through.

SUGAR FREE CHERRY & COCONUT FLAPJACK

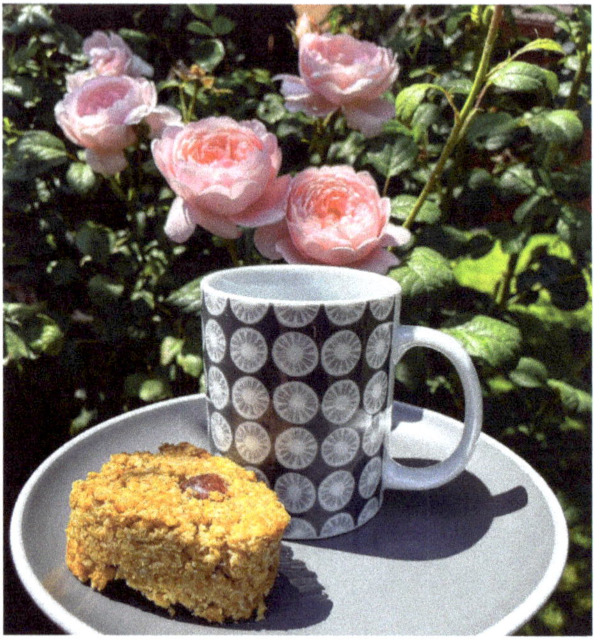

Ingredients

400g oats (gluten free oats for gf version!)
200g butter
100g desiccated coconut
Handful of cherries
200ml sugar free golden syrup

1. Pre-heat the oven to 180 degrees Celsius.
2. Melt the butter in a pan with the sugar free golden syrup, stirring continuously.
3. Remove from heat and add the oats, coconut and cherries to the melted butter and syrup. Mix well.
4. Press the mix into a lined tin and bake at 180 degrees for 25-30 mins until it is firm.
5. Remove from oven and chill the flapjacks for 3-4 hours before cutting.

SUGAR FREE JAM STARS

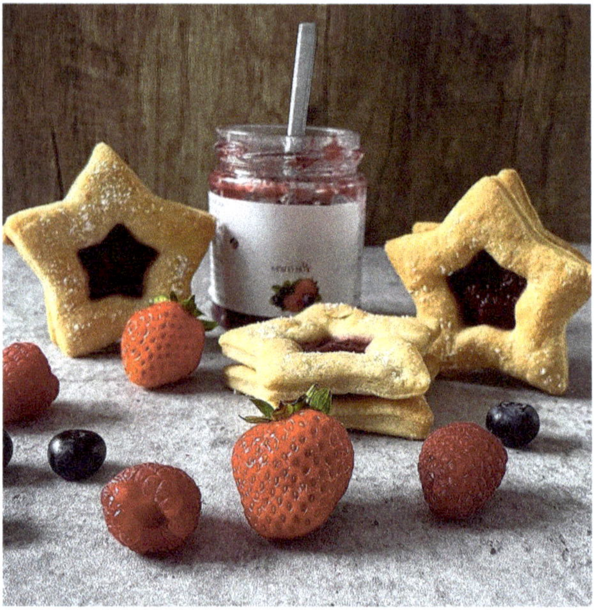

Pastry Stars

200g self-raising flour
(gluten free + 1tsp xanthum gum works too!)
100g butter

Filling

Sugar free jam

Decoration

Pinch of powdered sweetener

Pre-heat the oven to 180 degrees Celsius.

1. Use your fingertips to combine the flour and butter until it resembles breadcrumbs.
2. Add enough water to the mix to form a dough.
3. Roll out the dough onto a floured worksurface and, using a large and small star cutter, cut out your pastry stars – REMEMBER: You need the bottom star to have no hole in it so the jam doesn't fall out!!
4. Place the stars on a lined baking tray and cook for 10 mins or until golden.
5. Remove from the oven and let them cool completely.
6. Add a spoonful of sugar-free jam to the star (without a hole in) and then place another on top.
7. Once all of your stars are assembled, sprinkle on some sweetener.

NO ADDED SUGAR GLUTEN FREE APPLE TARTS

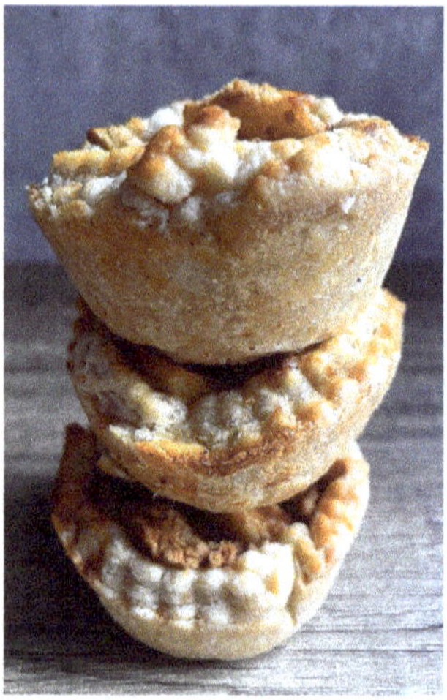

Makes 12 deep dish tarts

Pastry

125g gluten free self-raising flour
1tsp xanthum gum
60g butter or lard

Decoration

2 x gluten free spiced/ginger biscuits
1 x egg
1 x tbsp milk

Apple Filling

6 x small braeburn apples
(but any apple variety will do!)

Pastry

1. Rub together the butter, flour and xanthum gum until the mix resembles breadcrumbs.

Be careful not to overwork the pastry; if the mix is well-combined, stop rubbing!

2. Use water (add a little at a time!) to bring the mix together to form a ball.
3. Refrigerate for a minimum of 2 hours.
4. Once chilled, remove from the fridge and roll out to around 2mm thick.
5. Use a large round cutter to create the tart bases (measure your tin and always size up to make sure your bases fit easily!).

Pre-heat the oven to 180 degrees Celsius.

Filling

1. Peel and slice the apples and place them in a saucepan with two tablespoons of boiling water.
2. Stew them over a medium heat until soft.

Assembly

1. Use a 12-hole deep cupcake or muffin tin and place one tart base in each hole.
2. Use a tablespoon to evenly distribute your stewed apples between the tarts.
3. Crumble the spiced biscuits with your fingers and then place a little on the top of each tart.
4. Whisk the egg and milk with a fork and gently brush the top of the tarts.
5. Cook in the oven for 20-25 mins until golden brown.

LOW SUGAR TIRAMISU

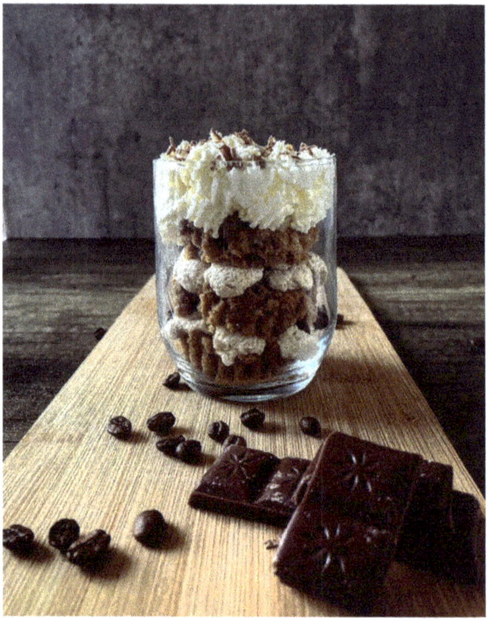

Coffee Sponge

100g self-raising flour (gluten free flour and 1tbsp xanthum gum works too!)
10g powdered sweetener
100g butter
2 eggs
1 tbsp milk
1 shot of espresso/2 tsp coffee granules dissolved in hot water

Cream Filling

250ml Double Cream
1 tbsp dissolved coffee granules/espresso
1 tbsp powdered sweetener

Chocolate Sponge

100g self-raising flour (gluten free flour and 1tbsp xanthum gum works too!)
10g powdered sweetener
100g butter
2 eggs
1 tbsp milk
2 tbsp low sugar cocoa powder dissolved in hot water

Decoration

Dark Chocolate Chips

Pre-heat the oven to 180 degrees Celsius.

Coffee Sponge

1. Mix together the butter and sweetener until light and fluffy using an electric mixer or whisk. The mixture should be almost white.
2. Add one egg at a time, with one tablespoon of flour. Mix until the egg is only just incorporated into the mix.
3. Remove the bowl from the electric mixer or transfer from using a whisk to a metal spoon. Fold in the remaining flour a third at a time.
4. Incorporate half the coffee mix/espresso and milk into the mix.

5. Transfer the mix to the tin and cook for 20 mins.
6. Insert a skewer into the middle of the cake to check it is cooked. Use foil to cover the top should it need a little longer and be turning too brown on top.
7. Leave to cool to room temperature.
8. Once cool, cut out rounds with a cutter to fit into your glasses for presentation. Alternatively, the top of the glass also acts as a great way to make sure you get the right size!
9. Pour the remaining coffee onto a plate and give both sides of the sponge a quick dunk.

Chocolate Sponge

1. Follow steps 1-3 above.
2. Incorporate the dissolved cocoa powder into the mix with the milk.
3. Transfer the mix to the tin and cook for 20 mins.
4. Insert a skewer into the middle of the cake to check it is cooked. Use foil to cover the top should it need a little longer and be turning too brown on top.
5. Leave to cool to room temperature.
6. Once cool, cut out rounds with a cutter to fit into your glasses for presentation. Alternatively, use the top of the glass as above.

Cream

1. Whisk the cream until it thickens. You should be able to still see the whisk's marks in the cream after you have stopped mixing.
2. Gently fold in the coffee and sweetener.

Assembly

1. Place one of the coffee sponges in the base of the presentation glass.
2. Pipe or spoon a layer of cream and sprinkle on some dark chocolate chips.
3. Place a chocolate sponge on top followed by cream with a few chocolate chips, alternate between coffee and chocolate sponges until the glass is full.
4. Pipe or spoon a final layer of cream on top and dust with cocoa powder or your chocolate chips!

NO ADDED SUGAR, GLUTEN FREE CHRISTMAS CHOCOLATE FRIDGE PUDDING

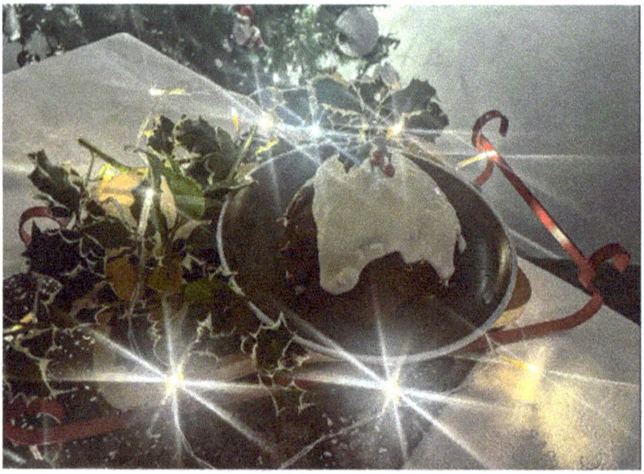

Ingredients

225g dark chocolate (over 70% cocoa)
225g butter (non-dairy alternatives work too)
2 eggs
10g powdered sweetener
50g mixed nuts (alternatively, you can use gluten-free biscuits crumbled)
100g salted popcorn

To decorate

50g Sugar free icing sugar/white choc whichever you prefer!

1. Melt the chocolate in a bowl over a saucepan of simmering water.
2. In a separate pan, melt the butter.
3. Beat your egg and sweetener together.
4. Add the melted butter to your egg mix.
5. Slowly stir in the melted chocolate.
6. Add your chosen fillings – nuts, biscuits, popcorn, dried fruit all work really well.
7. Line a pudding bowl with clingfilm and chill for at least 5hrs (best chilled overnight).
8. When ready to serve, tip out your pud and cover with white choc or use sugar free icing sugar mixed with water to make your topping.
9. Top with fresh holly for that festive feel!

NO ADDED SUGAR CHRISTMAS FUDGE

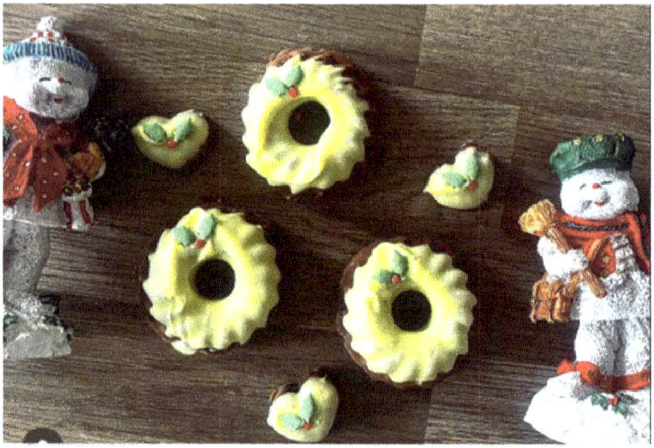

Ingredients

400g dark chocolate (over 70% cocoa)
1 x tin condensed milk
1 tsp mixed spice
1 tsp cinnamon
100g white chocolate

1. Melt the chocolate in a saucepan with the condensed milk, continuously stirring.
2. Add in your spices.
3. Melt your white chocolate and place a teaspoon in each of your mini bundt moulds.
4. Top up the moulds with your chocolate and condensed milk mix.
5. Leave to set in the fridge for at least 4hrs (best chilled overnight).
6. Remove your fudge and decorate as you wish!

LOW SUGAR GLUTEN FREE LEMON SHORTBREAD

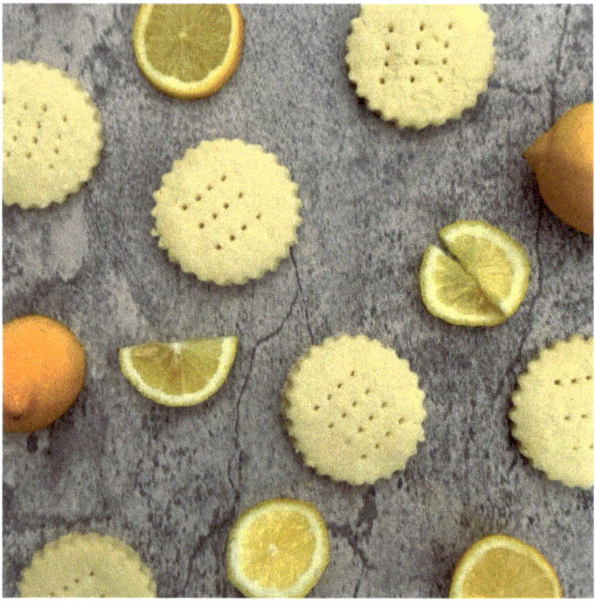

Ingredients

125g butter
15g caster sugar
2tbsp powdered sweetener
200g gluten free flour
50g cornflour
1tsp xanthum gum
Zest and juice of one lemon

1. Heat the oven to 150 degrees and line a baking tray with baking paper.
2. Mix together the butter, sugar and sweetener until combined.
3. Mix in the lemon juice.
4. Using a spoon, mix in the flour, xanthum gum and cornflour.
5. Add in the lemon zest.
6. Use your hands to bring it altogether.
7. Roll out the mix to approximately 1.5cm thick and use a cutter to make your shortbread into whatever shape you wish.
8. Cook for 18-20 mins.

SUGAR, GLUTEN & DAIRY FREE DECADENT CHOCOLATE MOUSSE

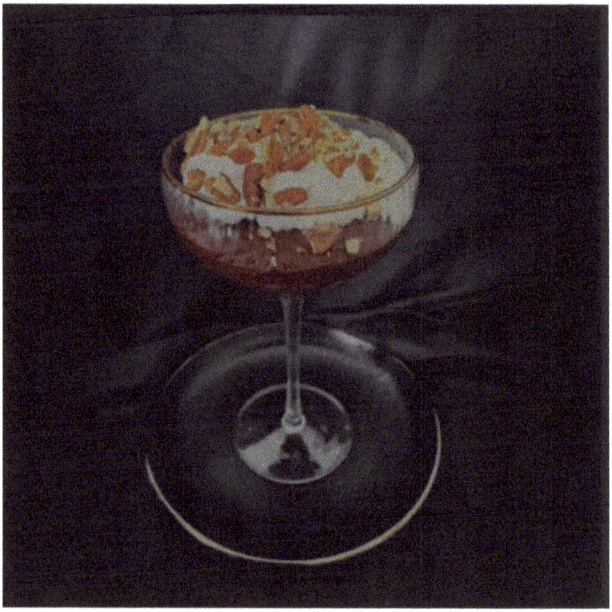

Ingredients

2 x ripe avocados
50g dark cocoa powder/low sugar cocoa powder
50ml almond milk
2tbsp powdered sweetener
Cream/nuts/berries – whatever you fancy for decoration!

1. Blend everything together in a blender.
2. Top with cream and your favourite toppings.
3. Chill for 20-30mins before serving.

LOW SUGAR, GLUTEN FREE BROWNIES

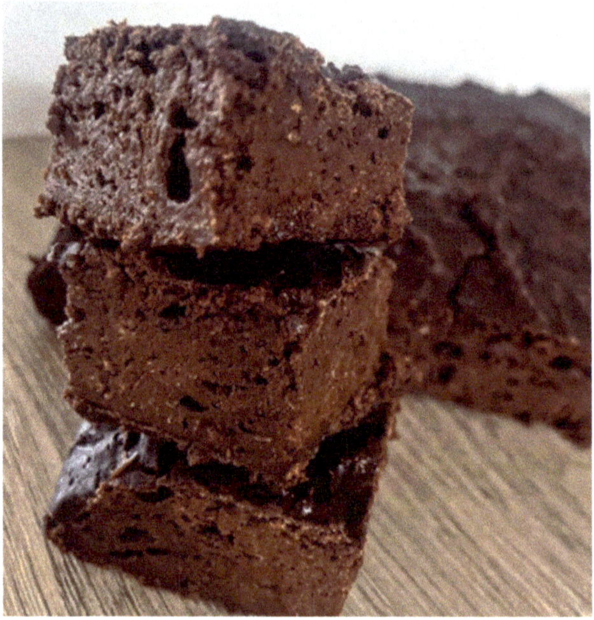

Ingredients

100g dark chocolate
3 large tablespoons Greek Yoghurt
10g powdered sweetener
100g gluten free self-raising flour
60g dark cocoa powder/low sugar cocoa powder
100ml skimmed milk

1. Preheat the oven to 180 degrees.
2. Melt your chocolate in the microwave, use short bursts and keep removing and stirring.
3. Leave your chocolate to cool for a minute or so before adding the Greek yoghurt and sweetener.
4. Mix until smooth.
5. Add your flour, cocoa powder and milk, mix again until smooth.
6. Transfer the mix to a lined 8 x 8 baking tray and cook for 25-30 mins until a skewer comes out clean.

NO ADDED SUGAR GLUTEN FREE SCONES

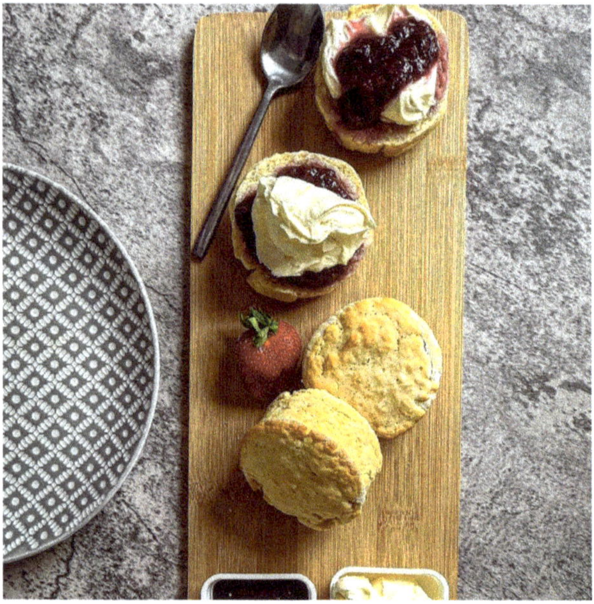

Ingredients

350g gluten free self-raising flour
1tsp gluten free baking powder
1tsp xanthum gum
1tbsp powdered sweetener
100g butter
200ml skimmed milk
2 x eggs

1. Preheat your oven to 200 degrees.
2. Combine the flour, baking powder, xanthum gum, sweetener and butter in a bowl. Use your fingertips to mix the ingredients until they resemble breadcrumbs.
3. Mix your milk and eggs together using a fork.
4. Add most of the mix to your dry ingredients, keeping a little leftover to brush the tops of the scones later.
5. Mix until it forms a dough.
6. Use your hands to press out the dough until its around 2cm thick.
7. Use cutters of desired size to create your scone.
8. Place your scones on a lined baking tray.
9. Brush the tops with the leftover milk and egg mix.
10. Bake in the oven for 12-15 mins until the tops are golden brown.
11. Serve with jam, cream, fresh berries or whatever you fancy!

www.ingramcontent.com/pod-product-compliance
Lightning Source LLC
LaVergne TN
LVHW050918210926
848482LV00012B/483